The Effective Management of Stress Urinary Incontinence

The Effective Management of Stress Urinary Incontinence

Edited by

Linda Cardozo FRCOG
Professor of Urogynaecology
Department of Urogynaecology, Kings College Hospital, London, UK

Dudley Robinson MRCOG
Consultant Urogynaecologist
Department of Urogynaecology, Kings College Hospital, London, UK

Andrew Miles MSc MPhil PhD
Professor of Public Health Sciences &
Editor-in-Chief, Journal of Evaluation in Clinical Practice,
Barts and The London,
Queen Mary's School of Medicine and Dentistry,
University of London, UK

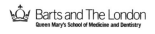

British
Society of
Urogynaecology

Association
for
Continence Advice

International
Continence
Society

AESCULAPIUS MEDICAL PRESS
LONDON SAN FRANCISCO SYDNEY

Published by

Aesculapius Medical Press (London, San Francisco, Sydney)
PO Box LB48, London EC1A 1LB, UK

British Library Cataloguing in Publication Data
A CIP catalogue record for this book is available from the British Library

ISBN: 1 903044 46 4

While the advice and information in this book are believed to be true and accurate at the
time of going to press, neither the authors nor the publishers nor the sponsoring institutions
can accept any legal responsibility or liability for errors or omissions that may be made.
In particular (but without limiting the generality of the preceding disclaimer) every effort
has been made to check drug usages; however, it is possible that errors have been missed.
Furthermore, dosage schedules are constantly being revised and new side effects recognised.
For these reasons, the reader is strongly urged to consult the drug companies' printed
instructions before administering any of the drugs recommended in this book.

Further copies of this volume are available from:
Claudio Melchiorri
Aesculapius Medical Press
PO Box LB48, Mount Pleasant Royal Mail Centre, Farringdon Road, London EC1A 1LB, UK

Tel: 020 7091 9671
Email: claudio@keyadvances.org.uk

Copy edited by The Clyvedon Press Ltd, Cardiff, UK

Typeset, printed and bound in Britain
Peter Powell Origination & Print Limited

Contents

Contributors

Paul Abrams MD FRCS, Professor of Urology, Bristol Urological Institute, Southmead Hospital, Bristol, UK

Kate Anders RGN BSc, former Senior Nurse Specialist, Department of Urogynaecology, King's College Hospital, London, UK

Duncan S. Barron BSc(Hons) MSc, Methodologist, HertNet/CRIPACC, University of Hertfordshire, Hatfield, Hertfordshire, UK

Gaia Bellini MRCOG, Clinical Research Fellow, The Warrell Unit, St Mary's Hospital, Manchester, UK

Donna Zimmaro Bliss RN, PhD, FAAN, Professor in Long-term Care of Elders, University of Minnesota School of Nursing, Minneapolis, MN, USA

Linda Cardozo FRCOG, Professor of Urogynaecology, Department of Urogynaecology, King's College Hospital, London, UK

Charlotte Chaliha MA MD MRCOG, Subspecialty Trainee in Urogynaecology, St. Mary's Hospital, London

Sinead Clarke-O'Neill RN MSc, Research Fellow, Continence and Skin Technology Group, University College London, UK

Kate Corlett MB ChB MRCGP, Hanscombe House Surgery, Hertford, Hertfordshire, UK

Alan Cottenden MA PhD MIPEM MIMMM CEng, Senior Lecturer in Medical Physics, Continence and Skin Technology Group, University College London, UK

Ayman Elnaqa MBBCh MSc MD MRCOG, Consultant Urogynaecologist and Obstetrician, New Cross Hospital, Royal Wolverhampton Hospitals NHS Trust, UK

Mandy Fader RN PhD, Reader, School of Nursing and Midwifery, University of Southampton, UK

Kathyrn Getliffe RN PhD, Professor of Nursing, Continence and Skin Technology Group, School of Nursing and Midwifery, University of Southampton, UK

Jeanette Haslam MPhil Grad Dip Phys MCSP RP, Clinical Physiotherapy Specialist in Women's Health, Honorary Visiting Lecturer, University of Bradford, UK

Hector H. Herrera MD MPH, Medical Officer, Urology and Lithotripsy Devices Branch (ULDB), Food and Drug Administration, USA

Vik Khullar AKC BSc MD MRCOG, Consultant Urogynaecologist, Department of Obstetrics and Gynaecology, St Mary's Hospital, London, UK

Mike Kirby MBBS LRCP MRCS FRCP, Director of the Hertfordshire Primary Care Research Network Consortium (HertNet), Letchworth; and Visiting Professor, CRIPACC, Faculty of Health and Human Sciences, University of Hertfordshire, Hatfield, Hertfordshire, UK

Matthew Parsons MRCOG, Consultant Gynaecologist, Birmingham Women's Hospital, Birmingham, UK

Jan Paterson RN PSM PhD, Associate Dean (Research) and Associate Professor, School of Nursing and Midwifery, Flinders University, Australia

Dudley Robinson MRCOG, Consultant Urogynaecologist, Department of Urogynaecology, King's College Hospital, London, UK

Chris Shaw PhD, Senior Research Fellow, University of Wales College of Medicine, Cardiff, UK

Mark Slack MB BCh MMed FRCOG, Consultant Gynaecologist and Lead Clinician, Urogynaecology, Addenbrooke's Hospital, Cambridge University Hospitals NHS Foundation Trust, Cambridge, UK

A. R. B. Smith FRCOG, Consultant Urogynaecologist, The Warrell Unit, St Mary Hospital, Manchester, UK

Sushma Srikrishna MRCOG, Urogynaecology Research Registrar, Department of Urogynaecology, King's College Hospital, London, UK

David Stott BA MSc DPhil, Statistician, Health Research and Development Support Unit, University of Hertfordshire, Hatfield, Hertfordshire, UK

George Szonyi FRACP FAFRM, Head, Geriatric Medicine, Royal Prince Alfred Hospital; and Director, Medical Services, Balmain Hospital, Sydney South West Area Health Service, Australia

Maria Vella MRCOG, Urogynaecology Research Registrar, Department of Urogynaecology, King's College Hospital, London, UK

Adrian Wagg MB BS FRCP, Consultant and Senior Lecturer in Geriatric Medicine, University College London Hospitals; and Associate Director, Clinical Effectiveness and Evaluation Unit (CEEU), Royal College of Physicians of London, UK

Ann R. Wagg BSc(Hons) MSc DPSN SRN, Senior Practice Nurse, Dr M O Wallis & Partners, Stevenage, Hertfordshire, UK

Judith Wardle PhD, Director, The Continence Foundation, London, UK

Mary Wilde RN PhD, Associate Professor, University of Rochester, New York, USA

Preface

Urinary incontinence (UI), the complaint of any involuntary leakage of urine, is a common and distressing condition which adversely affects quality of life. It can occur in a wide range of individuals of all ages and in both sexes with varying symptoms and severity. A study by the Continence Foundation of the UK has estimated that one in four women and one in nine men will suffer from urinary incontinence at some stage in their lives, thus representing a substantial section of Society. In the UK, significant progress has been seen in efforts to raise the public awareness of the effects of urinary incontinence and much of this work has been undertaken by the Continence Foundation, the Association for Continence Advice and Incontact. As a consequence of this work, it seems likely that help-seeking behaviour, and thus access to investigation and treatment, has been stimulated. Interestingly, the scale of the problem and its financial and social impact has only relatively recently become appreciated. Recent studies have shown that in the UK, for example, in excess of one-third of people aged 40 years plus (and thus approximately nine million people) are estimated to have a health care need for urinary storage symptoms and one-fifth (and thus approximately five million) are estimated to require health care related to urinary symptoms, with up to three million people being estimated to have unmet requirements. The nature and importance of what is therefore a major public health issue scarcely needs to be emphasized. Apart from a major impact on quality of life, clinically significant urinary storage symptoms have a substantial financial impact on the NHS constituting 1.1% of overall NHS spending for 1999/2000. The symptom of stress urinary incontinence (SUI) is the involuntary leakage of urine on effort, exertion or on sneezing and coughing, with the corresponding urodynamics observation being urodynamic stress incontinence, the involuntary leakage of urine during increased abdominal pressure, in the absence of detrusor contraction, noted during filling cystometry. SUI is the commonest type of incontinence, occurring as either pure SUI or as mixed urinary incontinence (MUI) and it is with the detailed study of SUI that this volume is concerned.

We have dedicated Part One of the book, through chapters 1–4, to a detailed study of the nomenclature and definitions of SUI, its epidemiology and pathophysiology and its impact on service use and treatment patterns. Writing in Chapter One, Abrams provides a concise account of the definitions employed in the study of lower urinary tract function and dysfunction collated by the International Continence Society. The importance of the ICS nomenclature, is, as the author points out, in the precision of its definitions, which allows accurate description of the patient's symptoms, signs and conditions and urodynamic assessment and therefore standardised communication between health care professionals. We move, in Chapter Two, to an epidemiological analysis of SUI contributed by Srikrisha, Vella and Cardozo. Prevalence estimates of UI vary as a function of the definition of incontinence employed and differ across the general population, among patients seeking help for other complaints in general practice or in gynaecology clinics and among other more selected groups of women. The estimates generated by population-based studies have sometimes included institutionalised women, consequently influencing prevalence estimation as well as distribution of severity, but in general terms, however, the prevalence of UI derived from epidemiological studies has shown variation ranging between 10 and 40%. The authors structure their chapter with a comprehensive examination of the potential risk factors for incontinence, including age, race, pregnancy and childbirth, menopause, hysterectomy, obesity, cognitive and psychiatric disorders, family history and genetics, abnormalities in collagen synthesis, occupation and lifestyle, exercise and smoking, providing an important synthesis of our knowledge of the epidemiology of SUI.

Having reviewed both nomenclature and definitions of UI within the context of SUI, and having considered our current knowledge of its epidemiology, we move in Chapter Three to a discussion of pathophysiology. As Slack and Elnaqa point out, it is unlikely that all cases of SUI have the same mechanism. Indeed, continence depends on the interplay between a variety of mechanisms, with urethral pressure, sphincteric dysfunction and associated pelvic floor damage all contributing to the pathophysiology of this condition. Over recent decades, a great deal has been published on the precise mechanisms which underlie the condition and many of the most important recent studies have been made possible by the revolution in diagnostic modalities which have provided important new insights into the function and dysfunction of the urethral continence mechanism, enabling theories to evolve from being purely anatomic to being both functional and anatomic. Slack and Elnaqa are clear that in clinical practice, multiple aspects, rather than a single aspect of the continence mechanism, are likely to be involved in symptomatic women and correction of one factor only may therefore prove insufficient to render the patient asymptomatic. Nevertheless, as the authors point out, as our knowledge of the neurocircuitry of the urethral continence mechanism expands, new modalities of treatment are becoming possible, giving both patient and clinician a wider choice of treatment options.

We conclude Part One of the volume with an essay by Shaw on the social disability of SUI and its impact on service use and treatment patterns. It is well accepted that SUI can result in considerable social disability and quality of life and that the impact on quality of life increases with the increasing severity of the condition, although this relationship is not a straightforward one. Indeed, women with relatively mild clinical symptoms sometimes report considerable impact, and vice versa, depending on their personal circumstances. As Shaw emphasises, the degree of social disability experienced by women with SUI is integral to their help-seeking decisions and their motivation to adhere to treatment plans. In this context, a proper assessment of the degree of disability is an essential component in the assessment of need and service planning. While acknowledging that the concept of quality of life and social disability is complex and that research assessing quality of life is open to a wide range of interpretation, the author nevertheless very usefully explores the relationship of social disability and quality of life impairments to women's illness behaviours and to health care professionals' treatment decisions, as well as presenting an overall view of the level of social disability resulting from SUI in the population. She is clear that help-seeking behaviour is not determined by symptoms alone, but rather by a complex set of factors which include symptom impact, coping resources, personal circumstances, awareness of the condition and treatment options. She thus concludes that there remains a need to improve patient knowledge and awareness in order to empower individuals to make appropriate health care choices and to enable them to self-manage symptoms in a more adaptive and effective manner.

We have dedicated Part Two of this volume, through chapters 5–7, to a detailed consideration of the evidence and opinion base for clinical assessment of SUI. Kirby and his colleagues, writing in Chapter Five, present a detailed discussion of the current knowledge base for medical assessment within the primary care setting. The authors agree with current guidelines, which place primary care in the forefront of the identification and management of urinary incontinence. As they point out, this benefits secondary care by ensuring that only patients who cannot satisfactorily be managed in primary care are referred. They are clear that successful management depends on an accurate and comprehensive assessment, followed by appropriate advice and follow-up. In Chapter 6, Anders discusses the evidence and opinion base for advanced nursing assessment in secondary care. For this author, a specialist nurse should be able to perform an array of investigations from simple urinalysis to cystometry and possibly videocystourethrography, with appropriate assessment prior to any therapy being of central importance if treatment is to be tailored to the individual sufferer of SUI and prove successful. Standard investigations will properly include a detailed history of the patient's condition, as well as full information regarding their medical, drug, surgical, obstetric and gynaecological history, with physical examination including vaginal examination to assess for prolapse and bimanual examination to exclude pelvic masses, given that uterine pathology, such as fibroids, can exacerbate SUI. A self-completed frequency volume chart allows an excellent measure of drinking, voiding and leakage patterns and should be sent before first consultation for at least 3 days. Investigative procedures inform uroflowmetry with post-micturition residual assessment either by in-out catheter or ultrasound; pad testing to quantify urinary leakage; and simple cystometry to exclude any abnormal detrusor activity. Other urodynamic investigations such as urethral pressure profilometry and ambulatory urodynamics are all increasingly performed by the specialist nurse, but are considered here in the chapter which follows.

There have been many different methods which have been proposed for the assessment of stress urinary incontinence in secondary care and it is to these that

Chaliha and Khullar turn in Chapter Seven. The first major category of such tests, as the authors describe, has used measures of urethral resistance to infer an assessment of urethral function relevant to stress incontinence. These include leak point pressure, where the pressures are measured in the bladder, vagina or rectum as the patient performs a manoeuvre to increase intra-abdominal pressure. Performing a Valsalva or cough can generate this increase in pressure; both produce different results in different women. Urethral pressure measurement has been used extensively to infer urethral function in relation to stress incontinence, and although successful in predicting the failure of incontinence surgery in the low pressure urethra, the test has not been useful in the diagnosis of urodynamic stress incontinence. Ambulatory urodynamics are frequently employed as second line investigations for the assessment of lower urinary tract disorders when laboratory urodynamics have failed to produce a diagnosis and have an established place in the investigation of stress incontinence. Further investigations are represented by imaging, which has been used to determine the pathology underlying the stress incontinence, mainly taking the form of 2D and 3D ultrasound in the measurement of bladder wall thickness and the assessment of urethral sphincter volume. There appear to be definitive differences between women with urodynamic stress incontinence and continent women with these tests. Lastly, the authors discuss the use of magnetic resonance imaging which, as they describe, has been used to study the pelvic floor and urethral sphincter, although with limitations due to, among other things, the lack of resolution. In conclusion, Chaliha and Khullar are clear that while interesting insights into the pathophysiology of stress incontinence have been obtained by these tests, none has as yet achieved proven diagnostic potential with the exception of cystometry.

Having considered the evidence base for clinical assessment in Part Two, we turn in Part Three of this volume, through chapters 8–11, to a review of the evidence base for clinical intervention. Behavioural modifications and physiotherapeutic interventions have been found to be effective in the treatment of stress urinary incontinence and it is to a detailed discussion of these that Haslam turns in Chapter Eight. Interventions should aim to both rehabilitate and strengthen the pelvic floor muscles in a functional way and also to ensure that lifestyle behaviour is favourable to success. However, prior to any physical examination it is essential, as she points out, to take a thorough history to ascertain any likely contributory factors. Pelvic floor muscle assessment will help in ensuring that a bespoke exercise programme can be prescribed specific to the individual's ability and this will underpin any other therapeutic interventions, but for those patients that are unable voluntarily to contract their pelvic floor muscles, greater involvement of the therapist is required to achieve therapeutic success. This additional therapy may involve the use of suitable neuromuscular electrical stimulation using appropriate parameters and some patients will respond to the use of other methods of biofeedback such as the use of a pelvic floor educator, vaginal cones, manometry or electromyography. Interestingly, physiotherapists have more recently started to use real time ultrasound as a method of biofeedback for rehabilitation purposes. Each of the methods that Haslam describes can be employed successfully when the therapist has undergone sufficient study and training and so the need to ensure adequate access of therapists to specialist training programmes remains of central importance to the success of physical therapy. Nevertheless, regardless of the type of therapy employed, motivation and compliance to therapy on the part of the patient is essential for any programme to be effective. The skilled therapist is therefore characterised as possessing not only research-based knowledge, but also the ability to harness it appropriately in the individual patient.

Containment products provide an alternative to surgery and medication for a large number of women with stress urinary incontinence and the types of products currently available may be broadly split into two categories: absorbent products and occlusive devices. In Chapter Nine, Fader and her associates present a thorough review of the containment products of use in the management of SUI, describing their different designs and characteristics. As the authors discuss, there have been relatively few formal studies of these products and those that have been conducted have a tendency to become quickly out of date as existing products are frequently discontinued and new products introduced. However, Fader and co-workers set out some broad conclusions from the published literature which they view of use as guides to practice. Female occlusive devices, for example, are very varied in design and although many have been introduced to the market, few of these products are still available. They may be subdivided into three categories: those that occlude at the external meatus, those that occlude in the urethra (intraurethral devices) or those that occlude via the vagina (intravaginal devices). Not all of these products have proved acceptable to women with SUI, but they have been observed to perform effectively in some women with evaluations yielding encouraging results. Unfortunately, because of the small market, many of the devices are no longer commercially available, so those who may have benefitted are denied the opportunity to try them.

A conservative approach is often justified in the management of SUI, especially if symptoms are only mild or easily manageable. Indeed, where a woman's family is incomplete or when symptoms manifest during pregnancy or immediately afterwards, surgery should be avoided and a range of other treatment options considered. Until very recently, there were no pharmacological interventions available for management, although various drugs such as alpha-1 adrenoceptor agonists, oestrogens and tricyclic antidepressants have all been used anecdotally in the past. There has thus remained a need for a safe, proven and effective drug (s) for use, where appropriate, and it is to a review of some of the new agents that Parsons, Robinson and Cardozo turn in Chapter 10, with specific discussion of the place of phenylpropanolamine, imipramine, oestrogens, desmopressin and duloxetine. Phenylpropanolamine (PPA) is given to provide positive reinforcement of alpha-adrenergic stimulation of the urethral sphincter that is normal in the filling phase of the micturition cycle. PPA has been shown subjectively to improve symptoms and is well tolerated in all of the small studies in which it has been used. Although there have been some objective changes in urodynamic variables, namely urethral closure pressure, there is no evidence that maximum urethral closure pressure (MUCP) is significantly correlated with subjective improvement. No patients in the studies were continent and dry after treatment with PPA and use of this agent has also been associated with an increased risk of stroke. For these reasons it is perhaps unsurprising that PPA has fallen out of favour in recent years. Only two small open studies of the use of imipramine have been undertaken, involving very small numbers of women. The efficacy was found to be of the order of 60%. On the basis of current evidence, its use cannot be advocated outside of clinical trials, especially in the light of problems with falls in the elderly. Oestrogens are known to have an important physiological effect on the female lower genital tract throughout adult life leading to symptomatic, histological and functional changes. Urogenital atrophy is the manifestation of oestrogen withdrawal following the menopause, presenting with vaginal and/or urinary symptoms. The use of oestrogen replacement therapy has been examined in the management of lower urinary tract symptoms as well as in the treatment of urogenital atrophy, although only recently has it been subjected to randomised placebo-controlled trials and meta-analysis. Oestrogen therapy alone has been shown to have little effect in the management of urodynamic stress incontinence. It has, however, been shown to improve outcome of treatment with PPA and future studies of duloxetine may study the effect of combination treatment in the same manner. Desmopressin represents a safe and effective treatment modality for the management of daytime urinary incontinence, by reducing urine output. Users are more likely to have no incontinence episodes in the first four hours after use and more likely to have a 'dry day', after use. Duloxetine represents the first pharmacological agent developed specifically for the treatment of stress urinary incontinence. It has been shown to be effective even with moderate and severe symptoms. The commonest side effect is nausea, but this is usually mild to moderate and transient. Discontinuation rates are very low, with nausea symptoms improving within a month or so. The onset of action is rapid with duloxetine – studies have demonstrated efficacy within a few weeks – and appears to be sustained. It may be that duloxetine used in combination with physiotherapy offers an excellent combination of more rapid improvement, sustained over time by improved pelvic floor muscle strength after physiotherapy. The mainstay of treatment for stress urinary incontinence remains physical therapy. However, for those women who fail to respond satisfactorily, duloxetine may offer an effective alternative to surgery and pelvic floor education in the management of women with moderate to severe stress incontinence.

Chapter 11, which concludes Part Three of this volume, focuses specifically on the assessment of surgical procedures to treat stress urinary incontinence in women and analyses the evidence in the medical literature to provide recommendations.

Levels of evidence and grades of recommendations are given according to the International Consultation of Urological Diseases (ICUD) system. Despite the number of operations described to treat stress incontinence and studies conducted, no consensus has yet emerged on which of them is the more effective. Indeed, a systematic review of the literature analysed the methodological quality of heterogeneous studies including randomised trials, non-randomised prospective studies and retrospective cohort studies evaluating surgery for stress incontinence and concluded that it was poor. In a particularly detailed contribution, Bellini and Smith review a range of current procedures, including anterior colporrhaphy, colposuspension, laparoscopic colposuspension, paravaginal repair, the Marshall-Marchetti-Krantz procedure, needle suspension, the pubo-vaginal slings, tension-free vaginal tape and injectable agents. They conclude that the evidence for any surgical procedure for the treatment of SUI is often limited by the poor quality of studies, small size of samples and different outcome measurements used. Only a few randomised trials have been published and even fewer have the power to determine the value of the procedure studies. Outcome measures employed, even when objective, often correlate poorly with patients' perceptions of their treatment, and peri-operative complications, postoperative pain and long term complications such as voiding dysfunction, detrusor overactivity and prolapse have not always been reported and studied in the necessary detail.

Part Four of this volume, the concluding Part, is concerned with a review of service development and evaluation. In the opening chapter of this section, Wardle discusses the concept of an integrated continence service and discusses the extent to which such systems of service organisation have been implemented into routine clinical practice within the UK. As she points out, the concept of integrated services was first expounded in detail in the Department of Health guidance document *Good Practice in Continence Services*, which built on earlier thinking on the clinical benefits of more comprehensive approaches to the provision of continence care, but a central difficulty has been the lack of availability of so-called 'best practice' models from which the continence community can learn. Wardle discusses the current status of development of integrated services by raising a series of questions. What, she asks, actually constitutes an integrated continence service? What progress has been made? What factors do services that are close to integration have in common? Additionally, she considers the range of barriers that act to prevent the achievement of an integrated service, among these being difficulties in persuading Trust boards to take an interest in effective continence care, problems in involving users and carers in the planning, provision and audit of services and in the general strategic development and operation of services. Care pathways that include assessment tools are an essential component of the primary and secondary elements of an integrated service and Wardle is clear on the importance of these mechanisms and the format that they should take. Similarly, she considers the importance of referral systems and the need to make these more 'logical' in the way that they operate, giving the example of a 'product champion', as it were, and the effects of such 'interventions' in facilitating quality improvements. Equally, effective systems to track the patient journey, so-called process mapping, are fundamentally important and should operate alongside the priovision of appropriate training to non-speclialists in the identification of continence problems in the first place. One of the remaining difficulties that is surely in need of urgent resolution is the correction of the current lack of convincing data that integrated contience services are overwhelmingly economically viable, cost-effective and in the interests of all patients and this is precisely where high quality audit data from methodologically rigorous evaluations will be of paramount importance.

With the broad considerations outlined by Wardle in mind, we move in the penultimate chapter, Chapter 13, to a review of Government targets, audit data and outcome indicators and their role in the measurement of clinical performance. Wagg frames his contribution against the backdrop of the Government encyclical *A First Class Service: Quality in the New NHS*, which set out a framework for quality improvement and fair access to services within the NHS. As he points out, clinical indicators and audit tools derived from practice guidelines were published for urinary incontinence in 1997 and 1998 and indicators such as these have been refined for clinical use over the years to allow specific judgements on the quality of services to be made. A variety of other sources of clinical knowledge on which indicators can be developed are additionally described as are the various reports and documents issued by the medical Royal Colleges and The Royal College of Nursing and the author looks forward, as do we, to the publication of NICE guidelines on the management of urinary incontinence, later this year, which will also, somewhat unusually, additionally consider issues relating to surgical competence in the field of continence care. As Wagg is clear, there has been a proliferation of practice guidelines for continence care in recent years and the NICE process may result in an useful formalization of these tools, with an associated development of quality measures with which to audit practice against the resulting guidance. An existing pilot study, published in the *Journal of Evaluation in Clinical Practice* and reviewed by the author, will undoubtedly go some way in informing the design of a more extensive national study, with direct effects on the effectiveness of clinical services and thus the quality of life of the patient.

It is to quality of life in the patient with lower urinary tract dysfunction that we turn in the final chapter of the volume, Chapter 14, by Robinson and Cardozo. As the authors point out, research has often concentrated on the prevalence, aetiology, diagnosis and measurement of urinary continence with little work being performed on the effects of this chronic condition or its treatment on quality of life. Over the past few decades, however, interest in the incorporation of patient assessed health status or quality of life measures into the evaluation of the management of urinary incontinence has increased significantly. The World Health Organisation has defined health as 'not merely the absence of disease, but complete physical, mental and social well being' and from a definitional point of view, 'quality of life' is widely understood to be measurable in terms of 'those attributes valued by patients including their resultant comfort or sense of wellbeing; the extent to which they are able to maintain reasonable physical, emotional and intellectual function, the degree to which they retain their ability to participate in valued activities within the family and the community'. This definition illustrates the multidimensional nature of quality of life and although highly subjective it is now acknowledged that it is as important as physical disease state in the management of women with lower urinary tract dysfunction. Consequently, and as Robinson and Cardozo point out, the success of treatment can no longer therefore be judged on clinical parameters alone and quality of life needs to be considered in both clinical and research settings. The authors usefully review a range of tools for the assessment of quality of life, including generic quality of life questionnaires, disease-specific quality of life questionnaires and the King's Health Questionnaire, all of which have been shown, to varying degrees, to be useful adjuncts in the investigation and management of women with lower urinary tract dysfunction complimenting standard investigations such as urodynamics and pad testing and representing important tools in both pharmacological and surgical trials, in clinical audit and in the assessment of new and established therapies.

We have aimed in the present text to provide a fully referenced clinical volume that is as succinct as possible, but as comprehensive as necessary. Consultants in urogynaecology, urology and integrated medicine and their trainees are likely to find the book of direct importance to their clinical practice and continuing professional development and we advance it specifically as an excellent tool for these purposes. We anticipate that the volume will also prove of considerable use to clinical nurse specialists in these fields and to general practitioners and their trainees and commend it also to the planners and commissioners of continence services as the basis for ongoing discussion and service development. In conclusion, we thank Eli-Lilly & Co Ltd and Boehringer-Ingelheim Ltd for a grant of unrestricted educational sponsorship which helped organise a major national symposium on stress urinary incontinence in association with the British Society of Urogynaecology, the International Continence Society, the Continence Foundation and the Association for Continence Advice at The Royal College of Obstetricians and Gynaecologists, London, at which synopses of the constituent chapters of this volume were presented.

Linda Cardozo FRCOG
Dudley Robinson MRCOG
Andrew Miles MSc MPhil PhD

London, July 2006

PART 1

Nomenclature & definitions, Epidemiology, Pathophysiology and Social Disability

Chapter 1

Stress urinary incontinence: nomenclature and definitions

Paul Abrams

The definitions used to describe lower urinary tract function and dysfunction, and the investigation methods, were collated by the International Continence Society (ICS) in 1988 (Abrams *et al*. 1988) and revised in 2002 (Abrams *et al*. 2002). In this book, the new definitions from 2002 are used.

In a survey of 2000 women in the Bristol UK area, 60% had some leakage according to the 2002 definition 'Incontinence as any involuntary leakage of urine' which is a definition suitable for epidemiological studies. Of the 60% who had some leakage, only a quarter had changed underwear, worn a protective pad or restricted social activities. Nevertheless, this means that 15% of women over the age of 20 are bothered by their urinary incontinence. This 15% would thus fit the previous ICS definition, which included the phrase 'also causing a social or hygienic problem', which encompasses the concept of leakage having a very significant impact on quality of life.

Figure 1.1 illustrates the pattern of incontinence in women according to type. Stress urinary incontinence (SUI) is the commonest type of incontinence, occurring as either pure SUI or as mixed urinary incontinence (MUI) together with urgency urinary incontinence (UUI). SUI can be a symptom, a sign seen on physical examination, or a condition when seen during urodynamic studies. The definitions are as follows:

- The symptom: Stress urinary incontinence is the 'the complaint of involuntary leakage on effort or exertion, or for example, on sneezing or coughing'.
- The sign: Stress incontinence is the 'observation of involuntary leakage from the urethra, *synchronous with* exertion/effort, or sneezing or coughing'. Stress leakage is presumed to be due to raised abdominal pressure.
- The condition: 'Urodynamic stress incontinence is noted during filling cystometry and is defined as the involuntary leakage of urine during increased abdominal pressure in the absence of a detrusor contraction.' USI is now the preferred term to 'genuine stress incontinence'. As the definition of USI implies, USI is diagnosed during the filling phase of pressure–flow studies.

In urodynamic stress incontinence (USI), urethral function studies are used, in some centres, to discriminate between intrinsic sphincter deficiency and bladder

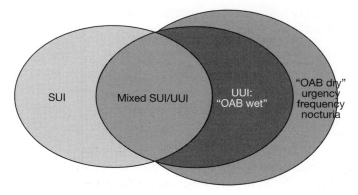

SUI: stress urinary incontinence
UUI: urgency urinary incontinence

OAB: overactive bladder is defined
as "urgency with or without urgency
incontinence, usually with frequency
and nocturia".

Figure 1.1 Storage symptoms and incontinence

neck/urethral hypermobility, the two principal causes of SUI. The two techniques most commonly used are defined as follows:

- 'The urethral closure pressure profile is given by the subtraction of intravesical pressure from urethral pressure.'
- 'Abdominal leak point pressure is the intravesical pressure at which urine leakage occurs due to increased abdominal pressure in the absence of a detrusor contraction.'

SUI may occur as part of mixed urinary incontinence (MUI) which becomes increasingly common in older age, primarily due to the increase in urgency urinary incontinence. Mixed urinary incontinence is defined as the complaint of involuntary leakage associated with urgency and also with exertion, effort, sneezing or coughing.

When UUI is seen during urodynamics it can then be termed 'symptomatic detrusor overactivity incontinence' or 'UUI due to detrusor overactivity'. The symptom Urgency Urinary Incontinence is defined as the complaint of involuntary leakage accompanied by or immediately preceded by urgency.

When assessing incontinence, a bladder diary is important as it allows the severity of the incontinence to be defined according to frequency and severity. Severity is most easily assessed by asking the patient to record pad usage and/or changes of underwear/clothing in the diary. The bladder diary gives the greatest amount of information of the three types of chart defined by ICS:

- Micturition time chart: this records only the times of micturition, day and night, for at least 24 hours.

- Frequency volume chart (FVC): this records the volumes voided as well as the time of each micturition, day and night, for at least 24 hours.
- Bladder diary: this records the times of micturitions and voided volumes, incontinence episodes, pad usage and other information such as fluid intake, the degree of urgency and the degree of incontinence.

In elderly persons, and particularly those who are frail, two other terms are useful when treatment is being discussed (Fonda & Adams, in press).

'Dependant Continence', meaning the situation where the individual would suffer a recurrence of incontinence if management was withdrawn. Examples would be; assisted toileting in the frail elderly and successful antimuscarinic treatment for urgency incontinence.

'Contained Incontinence', meaning that incontinence is controlled by being contained within an absorbent product or a collecting device. This term is preferred to the term previously used, 'social continence', which is felt to be misleading.

The importance of the ICS nomenclature is in the precision of its definitions, allowing accurate description of the patient's symptoms, signs and conditions, and urodynamic assessment. This ensures unequivocal communication between health care professionals.

References

Abrams, P., Blaivas, J. G., Stanton, S. L. & Andersen, J. T. (1988). The standardisation of terminology of lower urinary tract function. *Scandinavian Journal of Urology and Nephrology. Supplementum* **114**, 5–19.

Abrams, P., Cardozo, L., Fall, M., Griffiths, D., Rosier, P. & Ulmsten, U. (2002). The standardisation of terminology of lower urinary tract function: report from the standardisation sub-committee of the International Continence Society. *Neurourology and Urodynamics* **21**, 167–178.

Fonda, D., Abrams, P. (2006). Cure sometimes, help always – the continence paradigm. *Neurology and Urodynamics*, in press.

Chapter 2

Epidemiology of stress urinary incontinence

Sushma Srikrishna, Maria Vella and Linda Cardozo

Urinary incontinence (UI), the 'complaint of any involuntary leakage of urine' (Abrams *et al.* 2002; see also Chapter 1 of this volume), is a common and distressing condition known to adversely affect 'quality of life' (Kelleher *et al.* 1997). It may affect women of all ages and there is a wide range of severity and symptoms. The symptom of stress urinary incontinence (SUI) is the involuntary leakage of urine on effort, exertion, or on sneezing or coughing. The corresponding urodynamic observation is urodynamics stress incontinence, which is the involuntary leakage of urine during increased abdominal pressure, in the absence of a detrusor contraction, noted during filling cystometry (Abrams *et al.* 2002).

In epidemiological terms, *prevalence* is defined as the probability of experiencing a symptom, or having a condition or a disease within a defined population during a defined period, whereas *incidence* is the probability of developing the condition under study during a defined period.

Prevalence estimates of UI differ as a function of the definition of incontinence employed. These estimates also differ across the general population, among patients seeking help for other complaints in general practice or in gynaecology clinics and among other more selected groups of women. However, even across population-based studies using comparable definitions of incontinence, prevalence estimates vary (Herzog & Fultz 1990; Thom 1998). Some population-based surveys include institutionalized women, whereas others do not; this may influence prevalence estimation as well as distribution of severity.

In population estimates, the prevalence of UI varies from 10% to 40% (Hannestad *et al.* 2000) (Table 2.1). However, only 7–12% perceive it as a problem (McGrowther *et al.* 2001).

In the Norwegian EPINCONT community-based survey, 25% of all respondents had some urinary leakage, the prevalence being age dependent (Figure 2.1) (Hannestad *et al.* 2000).

Of the women studied: 50% complained of stress urinary incontinence; 11% complained of urge urinary incontinence and 36% complained of mixed urinary incontinence (Hannestad *et al.* 2000).

Smaller studies based on local communities support these high rates. At one general practice in Bristol, UK, the prevalence of UI was 53% (Harrison & Memel 1994). It is likely that most studies underestimate the prevalence of UI in populations owing to reporting bias and it is essential that this factor be addressed in all epidemiological surveys (Fultz & Herzog 2000).

The prevalence of all UI peaks at 45–55 years of age, dips slightly thereafter, then increases again after age 70 years (Thomas *et al.* 1980). It may be accompanied by an increasing incidence of overactive bladder symptoms, which have been shown to increase linearly with age (Milson *et al.* 2001).

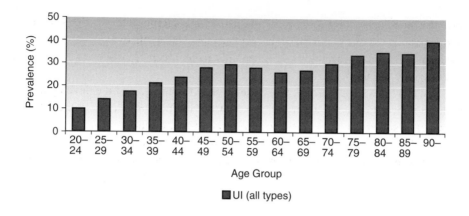

Figure 2.1 Prevalence of urinary incontinence (*n* = 27,936)

Table 2.1 Prevalence of any UI in the general population

Author	Year	Country	Response rate (%)	Age (years)	Number	Prevalence
Hunskaar *et al.*	2004	France	80	18+	3881	44
		Germany	59		3824	41
		Spain	64		6444	23
		Britain	45		2931	42
Blanco *et al.*	2003	Spain	82	40–65	485	15
Nygaard *et al.*	2003	USA	82	50–69	5701	16
Muscatello *et al.*	2001	Australia	68	41+	262	61
Hannestad *et al.*	2000	Norway	80	20+	27936	25
Chiarelli *et al.*	1999	Australia	48	18–23	14761	13
			54	45–50	14070	36
			41	70–75	12893	35
Milsom *et al.*	1993	Sweden	75	46–86	7459	21
Thomas *et al.*	1980	Britain	89	15+	7767	27

Types of urinary incontinence

The prevalence of different types of UI varies with age. Surveys suggest that mixed and urge urinary incontinence are more common in older women, whereas SUI is commoner in young and middle-aged women

Potential risk factors for incontinence

Age

Incontinence is not considered a normal part of the ageing process. However, there may be changes in the pelvic structure with age that may contribute to UI. In addition, medical conditions or diseases that disrupt normal continence may be more common in the ageing population.

Some studies have shown a significant link between age and the development of both urge incontinence and stress incontinence (Goldberg & Kwon 2003), whereas others have shown an association only with the former (Hannestad *et al.* 2000). In a large study of 842 women aged between 17–64 years, the prevalence rates of urinary incontinence increased progressively over seven birth cohorts (1900–1940) from 12% to 25%. As mobility and physical exercise decrease with advancing age, so does the prevalence of stress incontinence (Figure 2.2).

Race

Several studies have been performed examining the impact of racial differences on the prevalence of urinary incontinence in women. In general, there is evidence that there is a lower incidence of both urinary incontinence and urogenital prolapse in Black women. Studies in North America have found a larger proportion of White than African–American women reporting symptoms of stress incontinence (31% versus 7%), and a larger proportion were found to have demonstrable stress incontinence on objective assessment (61% versus 27%). Overall, white women had a prevalence of urodynamic stress incontinence 2.3 times higher than African–American women (Bump 1993). Stepwise logistic regression was used to compare risk factors for incontinence. Caucasian race was the most significant predictor of urodynamic stress incontinence (USI), and African–American race was the only significant predictor of detrusor overactivity (DO).

Pregnancy and childbirth

There is a relatively high prevalence of incontinence in pregnant women and, indeed, pregnancy is responsible for marked changes in the urinary tract. Consequently, lower urinary tract symptoms are more common and many are simply a reflection of normal physiological change. Urine production increases in pregnancy owing to increasing cardiac output and a 25% increase in renal perfusion and glomerular filtration rate.

Stress incontinence is the most common type of pregnancy-related urinary incontinence. Studies of UI in pregnancy have reported a prevalence of 32–64% for

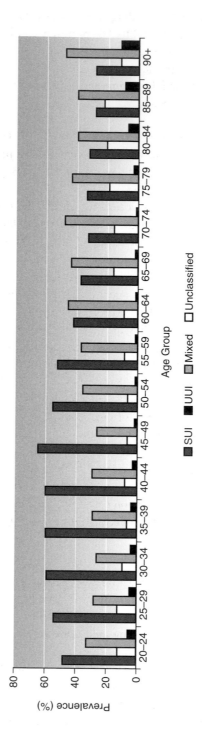

Figure 2.2 Age-dependent prevalence of incontinence

all UI and 40–59% for SUI (including mixed UI) (Stanton *et al.* 1980; Mellier & Delille 1990; Vikrup & Lose 1992). The prevalence is higher in parous women, although new onset UI is higher in primigravidae (Dimpfl & Hesse 1992; Marshall & Thompson 1998). During pregnancy, the prevalence of UI is low in the first trimester and then rises in the second and third trimesters. The severity of the incontinence also appears to increase during pregnancy (Burgio & Locher 1996; Goldberg & Kwon 2003).

UI in pregnancy is often a self-limiting condition (Vikrup & Lose 1992). However, some studies have shown that pregnancy UI is a predictor for post partum UI as well as a risk factor for incontinence for UI 5 years post-delivery (Hvidman & Folspang 2003; Burgio *et al.* 2003).

Several studies have shown a link between UI and parity (Holst & Wilson 1988; Sommer & Bauer 1990). Some authorities have found this relation to be linear, whereas others have demonstrated a threshold at the first delivery and some have shown that increasing age at first delivery is significant. A large Australian study has reported a strong relation between urinary incontinence and parity in young women (18–23 years), although in middle age (45–50 years) there was only a modest association and this was lost in older women (70–75 years) (Chiarelli *et al.* 1999).

Possible explanations for this link include pelvic floor laxity, impaired support to pelvic organs and damage to pudendal and pelvic nerves associated with childbirth. Vaginal delivery may predispose women to UI more so than delivery by Caesarean section, as shown in a recent study by Rortveit et al (2003). This study demonstrated a 10.1% incidence of any incontinence in nulliparous women, whereas the age-standardized prevalences were 15.9% in the Caesarean-section group and 21.0% in the vaginal-delivery group. Compared with nulliparous women, those who had Caesarean sections had an adjusted odds ratio for moderate or severe incontinence of 1.4. Only stress incontinence was associated with mode of delivery (Rortveit *et al.* 2003). Other factors, which may contribute to development of UI, include instrumental vaginal delivery, induction of labour, increasing foetal birth weight and prolonged labour (Thom DH, Van den Eeden 1997; Roe & Doll 1999).

Menopause

The urogenital tract and lower urinary tract are sensitive to the effects of oestrogen and progesterone throughout adult life. Lower urinary tract symptoms have been shown to be common in postmenopausal women attending a menopause clinic, with 20% complaining of severe urgency and almost 50% complaining of stress incontinence. There is inconsistent evidence linking menopause and loss of oestrogen to the development of UI (Rekers *et al.* 1999; Grady & Brown 2001). Oestrogen preparations have been used for many years in the treatment of urinary incontinence, although their precise role remains controversial. To clarify the situation, a meta-analysis from the Hormones and Urogenital Therapy (HUT) Committee has been reported (Grady & Brown 2001). Of 166 articles identified which were published (in English) between 1969 and 1992, only six were controlled trials and 17 were uncontrolled series. Meta-analysis found an overall significant effect of oestrogen therapy on subjective improvement in all subjects and for subjects with USI alone. Subjective improvement rates with oestrogen therapy in randomised controlled trials ranged from 64% to 75%, although placebo groups also reported an improvement of 10% to 56%. In uncontrolled series, subjective improvement rates were 8–89%.

Research also does not support lower levels of UI in women on HRT (Fabti *et al.* 1994).

Hysterectomy

The role of hysterectomy as a risk factor remains controversial. An oopherectomy at the time of hysterectomy puts a woman into a surgical menopause, which may indicate a hormonal mechanism in development of UI (Harrison & Memel 1994; Rekers *et al.* 1999).

Alternatively, there may be nerve damage post-hysterectomy or damage to the musculofascial attachments of the bladder neck to the pelvic sidewall (Alling Moller & Lose 2000). There have been different studies with conflicting results. In a survey of 3,896 women, those who had a hysterectomy were more likely to complain of UI than those who had not (21% versus 16%) (Milsom *et al.* 1993). However, several other studies have shown no such relation. Consequently, the effect of hysterectomy on the development of urinary incontinence remains controversial.

A relatively recent review of literature concluded that most studies did not demonstrate increased UI at 2 years post-hysterectomy (Fanti *et al.* 1994). The type of hysterectomy may also influence lower urinary tract function, although a randomised, double-blind trial comparing total and subtotal hysterectomy has shown no significant effect on frequency, nocturia, urge incontinence and stress incontinence (Thakar *et al.* 2002).

Obesity

Obesity has been linked with an increased risk of urinary incontinence (Burgio & Matthews 1991). Similar effects have also been reported after surgery for weight reduction (Bump *et al.* 1992; Subbak *et al.* 2005). Obesity has also been shown to be more common in women with an objective diagnosis of detrusor overactivity and urodynamic stress incontinence (Dwyer & Lee 1988). Overall there is good evidence to support the causal role of excess body mass in the development of urinary incontinence.

Cognitive and psychiatric disorders

In addition to the general population, urinary symptoms are frequently found in institutionalized women and those with psychiatric disorders. In 1995, a working party of The Royal College of Physicians reported that incontinence was suffered by: 15% of women living at home; 25% of women in residential care; 40% of women in nursing homes and 60% of women in long-term hospital care (Anonymous 1995).

Functional impairment, especially mobility limitations and sensory impairment, have been substantiated in several studies to be linked with UI (Aggazzoti & Pesce 2000). However, the exact relation between functional impairment and UI is still debated. UI may be a direct consequence of difficulty in getting to the toilet, a predictor of frailty or the consequence of an underlying systemic illness such as stroke.

Patients lacking mental orientation have a greater risk of UI than those with a normal mental status. Dementia increased the odds ratio of UI by 1.2 to 12.6% in one study (Fultz & Herzog 1999; Hunskaar & Borrie 1998).

Family history and genetics

There have been some studies that have shown evidence of a link between family history and SUI. At present, little is known about the genetic predisposition for UI. In one study of 161 monozygotic and 249 dizygotic twins, the inheritability was significant for urge although not for stress incontinence. In addition, studies indicate familial clustering: the relative risks for mothers, sisters and daughters of women with stress incontinence were 2.8, 2.9 and 2.3, respectively (Mushkat & Bukovsky 1996; Hamestaad & Lee 2004).

Abnormalities in collagen synthesis

There are data that link clinical, laboratory and genetic syndromes of abnormalities of collagen to pelvic organ prolapse and urinary incontinence (Al- Rawiz *et al.* 1982; Carley & Schaffer 2000). A recent study reported a differential gene expression in the pubococcygeus muscle related to actin, myosin and extracellular matrix proteins comparing women with prolapse to controls (Visco & Yuan 2003). We can hypothesise that these collagen abnormalities may also play a part in the development of incontinence.

Occupation and lifestyle

At present, there are few data about the effect of occupation on UI, although uncontrolled studies have suggested that heavy lifting predisposes to incontinence and urogenital prolapse. So far, only one study has examined female aircrew, for example. The authors found that 26% of 274 women complained of UI and that 18% complained of incontinence while at work. Although crew position affected the risk of incontinence, no other factors, including type of aircraft and performance of aircraft (military versus commercial), were significant (Fischer & Berg 1999).

Exercise

Although moderate cardiovascular exercise promotes general health and weight loss, heavy lifting predisposes to prolapse and incontinence (Davis 1996). Other studies have also shown that traumatic exercise may cause incontinence (Jorgensen *et al.* 1994).

Smoking

Smoking has been implicated as a risk factor in the development of UI although the exact mechanism is unknown. Smoking may contribute to chronic coughing which raises intra-abdominal pressure or impairment in collagen synthesis (Hannestad *et al.* 2000).

Conclusions

The causes of female urinary incontinence are multifactorial and although many common risk factors have been identified the impact of many more is less well documented (Table 2.2). Further epidemiological research should help clarify the importance of each which may improve primary prevention and subsequent treatment.

Table 2.2 Other risk factors for urinary incontinence

Lower urinary tract infection	Nocturnal awakening
Previous gynaecological surgery	Concomitant disease:
Childhood enuresis	Diabetes mellitus
Perineal trauma	Diabetes insipidus
Urogenital prolapse	Parkinson's disease
Pelvic radiotherapy	Dementia
Constipation	Stroke
Faecal incontinence	Depression
Diuretics (including caffeine)	Congestive heart failure

References

Abrams, P., Cardozo, L., Fall, M., Griffiths, D., Rosier, P., Ulmsten, U., Van Kerrebroek P., Victor A., Wein, A. (2002). The standardisation of terminology of lower urinary tract function: report from the standardisation committee of the International Continence Society. *Neurological Urodynamics* **21**(2), 167–178.

Aggazzoti, G., Pesce, F., Grassi, D., Fantuzzi, G., Righi, E., De Vita D., Santacroce, S., Artibani, W. (2000). Prevalence of urinary incontinence among institutionalized patients: a cross-sectional epidemiologic study in a midsized city in northern Italy. *Urology* **56**(2), 245–249.

Alling Moller, L., Lose, G., Jorgensen, T. (2000). Risk factors for lower urinary tract symptoms in women 40 to 60 years of age. *Obstetrics and Gynecology* **96**(3), 446–451.

Al-Rawiz, Z. S., Al-Rawi, Z. T. (1982). Joint hypermobility in women with genital prolapse. *The Lancet* **1**(8287), 1439–1441.

Anonymous. (1995). Incontinence. Causes, management and provision of services. A working party report of The Royal College of Physicians. *Journal of the Royal College of Physicians of London* **29**(4), 272–274.

Brown, J. S., Sawaya, G., Thom, D. H. Grady, D. (2000). Hysterectomy and urinary incontinence: a systematic review. *The Lancet* **356**(9229), 535–539.

Bump, R. C. (1993). Racial comparisons and contrasts in urinary incontinence and pelvic organ prolapse. *Obstetrics and Gynecology* **81**(3), 421–425.

Bump, R. C., Sugerman, H. J., Fantl, J. A., McClish, D. K. (1992). Obesity and lower urinary tract function in women: effect of surgically induced weight loss. *American Journal of Obstetrics and Gynecology* **167**(2), 392–397.

Burgio, K. L., Locher, J. L., Zyczynski, H., Hardin, J. M., Singh, K. (1996). Urinary incontinence during pregnancy in a racially mixed sample: characteristics and predisposing factors. *International Urogynecology Journal and Pelvic Floor Dysfunction* **7**(2), 69–73.

Burgio, K. L., Matthews, K. A., Engel, B. T. (1991). Prevalence, incidence and correlates of urinary incontinence in healthy, middle-aged women. *Journal of Urology* **146**(5), 1255–1259.

Burgio K. L., Zyczynski, H. Locher, J. L., Richter, H. E., Redden, D. T., Wright, K. C. (2003). Urinary incontinence in the 12-month postpartum period. *Obstetrics and Gynaecology* **102**(6), 1291–1298.

Carley, M. E., Schaffer, J. (2000). Urinary incontinence and pelvic organ prolapse in women with Marfans or Ehler Danlos syndrome. *American Journal of Obstetrics and Gynecology* **182**(5), 1021–1023.

Chiarelli, P., Brown, W. J. (1999). Leaking urine in Australian women: prevalence and associated conditions. *Neurourology and Urodynamics* **29**(1), 1–13.

Davis, G. D. (1996). Uterine prolapse after laparoscopic uterosacral transection in nulliparous airborne trainees. A report of three cases. *Journal of Reproductive Medicine* **41**(4), 279–282.

Dimpfl, T., Hesse, U., Schussler, B. (1992). Incidence and cause of postpartum urinary stress incontinence. *European Journal of Obstetrics, Gynecology, and Reproductive Biology* **43**(1), 29–33.

Dwyer, P. L., Lee, E. T., Hay, D. M. (1988). Obesity and urinary incontinence in women. *British Journal of Obstetrics and Gynaecology* **95**(1), 91–96.

Fantl, J. A., Cardozo, L. D., McClish, D. K. (1994). Oestrogen therapy in the management of incontinence in postmenopausal women: a meta-analysis. First report of the Hormones and Urogenital Therapy Committee. *Obstetrics and Gynecology* **83**(1), 12–18.

Fischer, J. R., Berg, P. H. (1999). Urinary incontinence in United States Air Force female aircrew. *Obstetrics and Gynaecology* **94**(4), 532–536

Fultz, N. H., Herzog, A. R. (2000). Prevalence of urinary incontinence in middle-aged and older women: a survey-based methodological experiment. *Journal of Aging and Health* **12**(4), 459–469.

Fultz, N. H., Herzog, A. R., Raghunathan, T. E., Wallace, R. B., Diokno, A. C. (1999). Prevalence and severity of urinary incontinence in older African American and Caucasian women. *Journal of Gerontology Series A: Biological Sciences and Medical Sciences* **54**, M299–M303.

Goldberg, R. P., Kwon, C., Gandhi, S., Akuru, L. V., Sorensen, M., Sand, P. K. (2003). Urinary incontinence among mothers of multiples: the protective effect of Cesarean delivery. *American Journal of Obstetrics and Gynecology* **188**(6), 1447–1450.

Grady, D., Brown, J. S., Vittighoff, E., Applegate, W., Varner, E., Snyder, T., HERS Research Group (2001). Postmenopausal hormones and incontinence: the Heart and Estrogen/ Progestin Replacement Study. *Obstetrics and Gynecology* **97**(1), 116–120.

Hamestaad, Y. S., Lie, R. T., Rortveit, G., Hunskaar, S. (2004). Familial risk of urinary incontinence in women: population based cross-sectional study. *British Medical Journal* **329**(7471), 889–891.

Hamestaad, Y. S., Rortveit, G., Sandvik, H., Hunskaar, S. (2000). A community-based epidemiological survey of female urinary incontinence: the Norwegian EPINCONT study. Epidemiology of incontinence in the county of Nord-Trondelag. *Journal of Clinical Epidemiology* **53**(11), 1150–1157.

Harrison, G. L., Memel, D. S. (1994). Urinary incontinence in women: its prevalence and its management in a health promotion clinic. *British Journal of General Practice* **44**(381), 149–152.

Herzog A. R., Fultz, N. H. (1990). Prevalence and incidence of urinary incontinence in community-dwelling populations. *Journal of the American Geriatric Society* **38**(3), 273–281.

Holst, K., Wilson, P. D. (1988). The prevalence of female urinary incontinence and reasons for not seeking treatment. *New Zealand Medical Journal* **101**(857), 756–758.

Hunskaar, S., Ostbye, T., Borrie, M. J. (1998). Prevalence of urinary incontinence in elderly Canadians with special association with dementia, ambulatory function and institutionalisation. *Norwegian Journal of Epidemiology* **8**(2), 177–182.

Hunskaar, S., Lose, G., Sykes, D., Voss, S. (2004). The prevalence of urinary incontinence in women in four European countries. *BJU International* **93**(3), 324–330.

Hvidman, L., Foldspang, A., Mommsen, S., Nielson, J. B. (2003). Postpartum urinary incontinence. *Acta Obstetricia et Gynecologica Scandinavica* **82**(6), 556–563.

Jorgensen, S., Hein, H. O., Gyntelberg, F. (1994). Heavy lifting at work and risk of genital prolapse and herniated lumbar discs in assistant nurses. *Occupational Medicine (Oxford, England)* **44**(1), 47–49.

Kelleher, C., Cardozo, L., Khullar, V., Salvatore, S. (1997). A new questionnaire to assess the quality of life of urinary incontinent women. *British Journal of Obstetrics and Gynaecology* **104**(12), 1374–1379.

Marshall, K., Thompson, K. A., Walsh, D. M., Baxter, G. D. (1998). Incidence of urinary incontinence and constipation during pregnancy and postpartum: survey of current findings at the Rotunda Lying-In Hospital. *British Journal of Obstetrics and Gynaecology* **105**(4), 400–402.

McGrowther, C. W., Shaw, C., Perry, S. I. *et al.* (2001). Epidemiology (Europe). In *Textbook of Female Urology and Urogynaecology* (ed. L. Cardozo & D. Staskin), pp. 21–35. Oxford: Isis Medical Media.

Mellier, G., Delille, M. A. (1990). Urinary disorders during pregnancy and post-partum. *Revue Francaise de Gynecologie et d'Obstetrique* **85**(10), 525–528.

Milson, I., Abrams, P., Cardozo, L., Roberts, R. G., Thuroff, J., Wein, A. J. (2001). How widespread are the symptoms of overactive bladder and how are they managed? A population-based prevalence study. *BJU International* **88**(7), 807.

Milsom, I., Ekelund, P., Molander, U, Arvidsson, L., Areskoug, B. (1993). The influence of age, parity, oral contraception, hysterectomy and menopause on the prevalence of urinary incontinence in women. *Journal of Urology* **149**(6), 1459–1462.

Muscatello, D., Rissel, C., Szonyi, G. (2001). Urinary symptoms and incontinence in an urban community: prevalence and associated factors in older men and women. *Internal Medicine Journal* **31**(3), 115–160.

Mushkat, Y., Bukovsky, I, Langer, R. (1996). Female urinary stress incontinence – does it have familial prevalence? *American Journal of Obstetrics and Gynecology* **174**(2), 617–619.

Nieto Blanco, E., Camacho Perez J. Davila Alvarez, V., Ledo Garcia, M. P., Moriano Bejar, P., Perez Lorente, M., Serrano Molina, L., Fonseca Redondo, B. (2003). *Aten Primaria* **32**(7),410–414.

Nygaard, I., Turvey, C., Burns, T. L., Crischilles, E., Wallace, R. (2003). Urinary incontinence and depression in middle aged United States women. *Obstetrics and Gynecology* **101**(1), 149–156.

Rekers, H., Drogendik, A. C., Valkenburg, H. A., Riphagen, F. (1992). The menopause, urinary incontinence and other symptoms of the genito-urinary tract. *Maturitas* **15**(2), 101–111.

Roe, B., Doll, H. (1999). Lifestyle factors and continence status: comparison of self-report data from a postal survey in England. *Journal of Wound, Ostomy and Continence Nursing* **26**(6), 312–313, 315–319.

Rortveit, G., Dalveit, A. K., Hannestad, Y. S., Hunskaar, S. (2003). Urinary incontinence after vaginal delivery or caesarean section. *New England Journal of Medicine* **348**(10), 900–907.

Sommer, P., Bauer, T., Nielson, K. K., Kristensen, E. S., Hermann, G. G., Steven, K., Nordling, J. (1990). Voiding patterns and prevalence of incontinence in women. A questionnaire survey. *British Journal of Urology* **66**(1), 12–15.

Stanton, S. L., Kerr-Wilson, R. Harris, V. G. (1980). The incidence of urological symptoms in normal pregnancy. *British Journal of Obstetrics and Gynaecology* **87**(10), 897–900.

Subak, L. L., Whitcomb, E., Shen, H., Saxon, J., Vittinghoff, E., Brown, J. S. (2005). Weight loss: a novel and effective treatment for urinary incontinence. *Journal of Urology* **174**(1), 190–195.

Thakar, R., Ayers, S., Clarkson, P., Stanton, S., Mayonda, I. (2002). Outcomes after total versus subtotal abdominal hysterectomy. *New England Journal of Medicine* **347**(17), 1318–1325.

Thom, D. H., van den Eeden, S. K., Brown, J. S. (1997). Evaluation of parturition and other reproductive variables as risk factors for urinary incontinence in later life. *Obstetrics and Gynecology* **90**(6), 983–989.

Thomas, T. M., Plymat, K. R., Blannin, J., Meade, T. W. (1980). Prevalence of urinary incontinence. *British Medical Journal* **281**(6258), 1243–1245.

Thom, D. (1998). Variation in estimates of urinary incontinence prevalence in the community: effects of differences in definition, population characteristics and study type. *Journal of the American Geriatrics Society* **46**(4), 473–480.

Vikrup, L., Lose, G. Rolff, M., Barfoed, K. (1992). The symptom of stress incontinence caused by pregnancy or delivery in primiparas. *Obstetrics and Gynecology* **79**(6), 945–949.

Visco, A. G., Yuan, L. (2003). Differential gene expression in pubococcygeus muscle from patients with pelvic organ prolapse. *American Journal of Obstetrics and Gynecology* **189**(1), 102–112.

Chapter 3

Pathophysiology of stress urinary incontinence

Mark Slack and Ayman Elnaqa

Introduction

It is unlikely that all cases of stress urinary incontinence (SUI) have the same mechanism. Continence depends on the interplay between a variety of mechanisms. Urethral pressure, sphincteric dysfunction and associated pelvic floor damage all contribute to SUI pathophysiology. In order to manage SUI optimally, a thorough understanding of these factors is necessary.

The exact cause of SUI is complex and remains elusive. Currently, the pathophysiology of SUI is considered to be multifactorial and theories regarding it have been evolving since the late eighteenth century. Changes in understanding were driven by the discovery of new diagnostic modalities that gave insight into the function of the bladder.

Mann's textbook *American System of Gynaecology* proposed an anatomic basis. He suggested that a urethrocele was a 'dislocation of the urethra' secondary to prolapse of the anterior vaginal wall and only mentioned that incontinence was a common occurrence as an afterthought (Cundiff 2004).

In 1914, Kelly (Kelly & Dumm 1914) used his cystoscope to describe SUI and attributed SUI to 'vesical neck funnelling' secondary to loss of elasticity or normal tone of the urethral sphincter. His hypothesis about the involvement of sphincter tone was the predecessor of future functional theories of SUI pathophysiology.

In 1923, Bonney (Bonney 1923) made a clear description of the relationship between exertion and incontinence and the role of childbearing in the epidemiology of SUI. His paper sought to explain the pathophysiology of SUI in terms of failure of anatomic support by which sagging of the pubocervical muscle sheet interfered with the sphincter mechanism. His theory became the foundation of the subsequent theories attributing SUI to anatomic failure.

In 1937, Stevens and Smith (Stevens & Smith 1937), using a watch-chain cystogram, described 'funnelling of the bladder floor toward the urethra' and flattening of the urethrovesical angle. They hypothesised that the anatomic abnormalities were a reflection of a weak sphincter. This concept was almost certainly influenced by the writings of Kennedy (Kennedy 1937) in 1937 who suggested injury to the urethral sphincter and the innervation as possible causes of SUI.

Pressure transmission theories

Barnes (Barnes 1940) used manometry and watch-chain cystography to study urethral function. He recognised that urethral damage could be direct to the sphincter or indirectly to the surrounding urethral structures. He further concluded that 'it would appear that incontinence could result from: (a) an increase in urinary expulsive forces or intravesical pressure; (b) a lowering of the powers of resistance or urethral sphincter action, or: (c) a combination of (a) and (b).'

Enhörning (Enhörning 1961) developed a urethral catheter with two pressure transducers 5 cm apart, which permitted simultaneous measurement of vesical and urethral pressures. Using this apparatus, he showed that equal rise in vesical and urethral pressure was due to transmission of intra-abdominal pressure to the bladder and the part of the proximal urethra above the pelvic floor. The transmitted intra-abdominal pressure maintained continence by augmenting the pressure resulting from sphincteric function. Conversely, 'In cases of stress incontinence this upper part of the urethra is often relaxed into a funnel and has then functionally become part of the bladder. If muscles with sphincteric function do not compensate for the incompleteness in transmittance of intra-abdominal pressure to the remaining lower part of the urethra, closure pressure decreases during a cough and incontinence may be manifested.' (Enhörning 1961).

As urodynamic studies became more sophisticated, doubt was placed on the transmission theory and attention was focused on abnormalities in urethral closure pressure and urethral length.

Sphincteric dysfunction theories

Snooks and colleagues (Snooks *et al.* 1985) used nerve conduction techniques to demonstrate prolonged conduction in the pudendal nerve thus suggesting a neurogenic role in the aetiology of SUI. This work was supported by the work of Smith and colleagues (Smith *et al.* 1989) who demonstrated denervation injury to both the striated urethral muscle and the pelvic floor musculature in women with SUI.

For those attempting to find an universal theory for the aetiology of SUI, the neurogenic theory did not fit easily with the pressure transmission theory. As a result, a subset of SUI was suggested to result from urethral sphincter deficiency. Because of the inherent difficulties in measuring urethral pressure, a variety of urodynamic definitions arose to describe this entity (Lose 2001) A maximum urethral closure pressure (MUCP) of < 20 cm H_2O or leak point pressure (LPP) < 65 cm H_2O, are the levels below which the diagnosis is made. Questions have been raised about the relationship of these measurements to severity and of the correlation between the two measurements. The same authors concluded that each measurement measures something different about the urethral function (Slack *et al.* 2004).

The division of the pathophysiology of SUI into urethral support failure and urethral sphincteric failure seemed to validate both the anatomic and functional theories by making them mutually exclusive. Complex classifications arose from the theories in an attempt to define groups of patients best treated with specific surgical techniques. On the basis of limited information, surgeons recommended one of the variations of retropubic urethropexy for women with urethral support failure, while reserving the suburethral sling procedures for patients with sphincteric failure (Cundiff 2004).

In recent times, with the introduction of new operations, surgeons seem to have given up attempts to develop subsets. This is partly because of the perceived success of the new slings and because of concern over the predictive validity of urodynamic tests. However, as these operations still have significant failure rates, efforts should be concentrated on gaining a better understanding of continence mechanisms and, by so doing, enhancing the development of better tests for diagnosis.

Continence mechanism during stress

Urethra

To understand the urethral role in maintaining continence during stress, we have to overview the functional anatomy of the urethra.

The urethra is a complex tubular organ, 3–4 cm long, extending below the bladder. It begins at the internal urethral meatus and terminates in the vestibule at the external meatus. The upper one-third is separable from the vagina, but the lower portion, as a reflection of its embryological derivation, is fused and embedded within the substance of the vagina.

The function of the urethra differs along its length. To facilitate understanding at the different portions it helps to divide the organ into fifths (DeLancey 1986).

Striated urogenital sphincter

The outer layer of the urethra is formed by the muscle of the striated urogenital sphincter (Figures 3.1, 3.2) which is found from about 20% to 80% of the total urethral length. In its upper two-thirds, the sphincter fibres lie in a primarily circular orientation; distally, they encircle the vaginal wall as the *urethrovaginal sphincter* and extend along the inferior pubic ramus above the perineal membrane (urogenital diaphragm) as the *compressor urethrae*.

This muscle is composed largely of slow-twitch muscle fibres (type I) that exert a constant tone upon the urethral lumen. The somatic innervation of the external urethral sphincter is from the pudendal nerve (S2, S3, S4). During bladder filling, pudendal motor neurones are activated by vesical afferent input (Park *et al.* 1997). During micturition these motor neurones are reciprocally inhibited (de Groat *et al.* 1993). In addition, voluntary muscle activation increases urethral resistance during events that require rapid, albeit short-lived, increases in urethral closure pressure. In the distal urethra, this striated muscle compresses the urethra from above; proximally, it constricts the lumen. Studies of skeletal muscle blockade suggest that

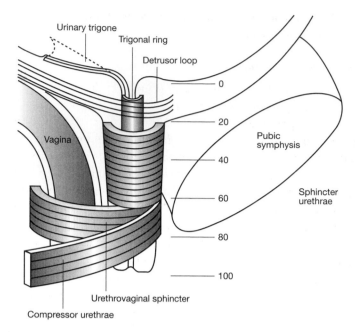

Figure 3.1 Schematic diagram of the striated urogenital sphincter muscle and trigonal musculature within the bladder base and urethra (cut in sagittal section). The ruler indicates the locations of structures along the urethral length. (DeLancey 1986).

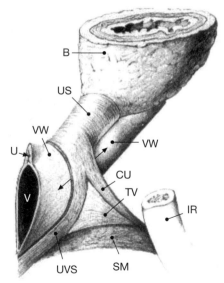

Figure 3.2 Striated urogenital sphincter muscle seen from below after removal of the pubic bones. US, urethral sphincter; UVS, urethrovaginal sphincter; CU, compressor urethrae; B, bladder; TV, transverse vaginal muscle; SM, smooth muscle; U, urethra; VW, vaginal wall; V, vagina; IR, ischiopubic ramus. (DeLancey 1986).

this muscle is responsible for approximately one-third of resting urethral closure pressure (Heesakkers & Gerretsen 2004).

Urethral smooth muscle

The smooth muscle of the urethra is contiguous with that of the trigone and detrusor. It has an inner longitudinal layer and a thin outer circular layer, with the former being by far the more prominent of the two. The layers lie inside the striated urogenital sphincter muscle, and are present throughout the upper four-fifths of the urethra. The excitatory pathways that maintain continence originate in sympathetic preganglionic neurones. The peripheral efferent pathways pass through the sympathetic chain ganglia to the inferior mesenteric ganglia and then via the hypogastric nerves to the pelvic ganglia (Kihara & de Groat 1997). Excitation of bladder neck and urethral smooth muscle via sympathetic innervation is mediated by activation of alpha-1 adrenergic receptors. This is mediated reflexly during afferent activity induced by distension of the urinary bladder. This reflex is inhibited during micturition. The smooth muscle also has muscarinic, cholinergic and purinergic influences, but noradrenaline from sympathetic innervation is primarily responsible for urethral smooth muscle contraction during the storage phase of the micturition cycle. The innervation and longitudinal orientation of most of the muscle fibres suggest an active role to shorten and funnel the urethra during voiding. The configuration of the circular muscle suggests a role in constricting the lumen (DeLancey 1994).

Submucosal vasculature

Within the urethra there is a well-developed vascular plexus that shows the presence of several specialised types of arteriovenous anastomoses. They have been shown to inflate and deflate and as such can assist in forming a watertight closure of the mucosal surfaces. Occlusion of the arterial inflow to these venous reservoirs has been shown to influence urethral closure pressure. These appear to be hormone sensitive, which may help to explain some individuals' response to oestrogen supplementation (DeLancey 1994). The percentage contribution to the incontinence mechanism is difficult to determine.

Mucosa

The mucosal lining of the urethra is continuous above with the transitional epithelium of the bladder. The mucosa is hormonally sensitive and undergoes significant change depending on its state of stimulation. The mucosa is tightly co-apted and certainly contributes to a watertight seal.

Connective tissue

In addition to the contractile and vascular tissue of the urethra, there are considerable quantities of connective tissue interspersed within the muscle and the submucosa.

As they are relatively inert and have little or no neurological function it is difficult to devise experiments to establish their precise role in the continence mechanism (DeLancey 1994).

Vesical neck

The term 'vesical neck' is both a regional and a functional one. It is the area at the base of the bladder where the urethra passes through the bladder wall. Therefore, it is sometimes considered as part of the bladder musculature, but it also contains the urethral lumen studied during urethral pressure profilometry.

The vesical neck has come to be considered separately from the bladder and urethra because it has unique functional characteristics. Specifically, sympathetic denervation or damage of this area results in its remaining open at rest; when this happens in association with stress incontinence, simple urethral suspension is often ineffective in curing this problem (DeLancey 1994).

Urethral and anterior vaginal wall support

The anatomic position and mobility of the bladder and urethra have long been recognised to have an important role in determining continence. The pelvic floor musculature and endopelvic fascia are responsible for the position and fixation of these organs (DeLancey 1994). Ultimately, the support is provided by the attachment of these structures to the bony pelvis or its muscles. The endopelvic fascia attaches the uterus and vagina to the pelvic wall. DeLancey divided the supports of the pelvic organs into three compartments. Level I supports the upper one-third of the vagina and the uterus. The fascia here is contiguous with the uterosacral and cardinal ligaments. These fibres are suspensory and run in a nearly vertical direction from a broad base of attachment over the piriformis, the sacroiliac joint and the ala of the sacrum. Level II provides most of the support of the middle of the vagina and with it the support of the bladder and rectum. Here, the endopelvic fascia attaches to the side wall of the pelvis. It attaches along the arcus tendineus fascia pelvis (the white line) which runs from the symphysis pubis to the ischial spine. This level is crucial to the support of the urethra as it provides posterior support. The posterior support of the bladder and urethra can suffer damage during childbirth or secondary to loss of muscle support. In level III the tissues are fused to the surrounding structures. This level is the one least likely to suffer damage.

Current theories

Taking the above into account it becomes obvious that urethral closure pressure results from the smooth muscle component, the external urethral sphincter and a non-muscular component including the vascular plexus and mucosal coaption. All provide a similar contribution to continence. In addition it is obvious that loss of urethral support will contribute to loss of continence. Finally it is increasingly becoming obvious that central nervous system dysfunction can provide yet another explanation for loss of the normal continence mechanism.

In 1996, DeLancey (DeLancey 1996) proposed a consolidated theory of SUI. Using anatomic research, he hypothesised that the pubocervical fascia and pelvic muscles provide hammock-like support for the vesical neck creating a backboard for compression of the proximal urethra during episodes of increased intra-abdominal pressure. Loss of this support would compromise equal transmission of intra-abdominal pressure. This part of DeLancey's theory combines the theories of Bonney and Enhörning. However, his theory also accounts for neuromuscular dysfunction. DeLancey's anatomic observations showed a connection of the pubocervical fascia with the insertion of the levator ani muscles at the symphysis pubis. He hypothesised that this connection with the levator ani muscles permits active elevation of the vesical neck during contraction of the levator ani muscles. This part of the theory provides a mechanism for SUI due to neuromuscular injury.

Petros and Ulmsten (Petros & Ulmsten 1990) proposed the integral theory of urinary incontinence. They argued that stress and urge symptoms both derive, for different reasons, from anatomic laxity in the anterior vaginal wall. The laxity may be caused by defects in the vaginal wall itself or in the ligaments and muscles that support it. According to this theory, the vaginal wall has a structural function that prevents SUI by transmitting the muscle movements involved in bladder neck opening and closing, as well as a function that prevents urgency by supporting hypothesised stretch receptors located in the proximal urethra and bladder neck. There is little support for this concept in the physiological literature. This theory is probably an oversimplification which ignores current physiological understanding and is aimed at supporting the midurethral tape as the solution for the treatment of SUI.

Recent investigations of urethral sphincteric dysfunction

Ongoing research is providing further insight into urethral sphincteric function. Lose (Lose & Colstrup 1991) showed a significant decrease in power generation at the bladder neck and midurethra in the subjects with SUI, suggesting the presence of an active closure mechanism in the midurethra.

Kamo and colleagues (Kamo et al. 2003) demonstrated a similar dynamic closure. They are suggesting that the midurethra closes by an active contraction mechanism in addition to the passive mechanism of the proximal urethra. Moreover, in the midurethra, the active urethral closure pressure was not related to the magnitude of bladder response, and the urethral response began before the bladder response.

Thind and Lose (Thind & Lose 1994) evaluated urethral pressure and power in ten healthy women before and after pudendal blockade. The investigators hypothesised that pudendal injury with resulting external urethral sphincter weakness has pathophysiological significance in SUI. This work is supported by similar findings following pudendal nerve injury in rats (Kerns et al. 2000).

There has also been significant progress in elucidating the neurotransmitters responsible for urethral function. The external urethral sphincter reflexes are enhanced by serotonin agonists and depressed by serotonin antagonists (Danuser & Thor 1996; de Groat *et al.* 1999), suggesting that the descending serotonergic pathways are responsible for the spinal cord circuitry controlling the closure mechanism of the external urethral sphincter.

Conclusion

Over the past few decades, much has been discovered about the pathophysiology of SUI. The revolution in diagnostic modalities has provided new insight into the function and dysfunction of the urethral continence mechanism and theories have evolved from being purely anatomic to being both functional *and* anatomic. In clinical practice, multiple aspects rather than a single aspect of the continence mechanism are probably involved in symptomatic women; consequently, correction of one of the injuries may not be sufficient to render the patient asymptomatic. As our knowledge of the neurocircuitry of the urethral continence mechanism expands, new modalities of treatment are becoming possible, giving both the patient and clinician a wider choice of treatment options.

References

Barnes, A. (1940). A method for evaluating the stress of urinary incontinence. *American Journal of Obstetrics and Gynecology* **40**, 381–390.

Bonney, V. (1923). On diurnal incontinence of urine in women. *Journal of Obstetrics and Gynaecology of the British Empire* **30**, 358–365.

Cundiff, G. W. (2004). The pathophysiology of stress urinary incontinence: a historical perspective. *Reviews in Urology* **6** (suppl 3), S10–S18.

Danuser, H. & Thor, K. B. (1996). Spinal 5-HT2 receptor-mediated facilitation of pudendal nerve reflexes in the anaesthetized cat. *British Journal of Pharmacology* **118**, 150–154.

de Groat, W. C., Booth, A. M. & Yoshimura, N. (1993). Neurophysiology of micturition and its modification in animal models of human disease. In *The Autonomic Nervous System*, vol. III (ed. C. A. Maggie), pp 227–289. London: Harwood.

de Groat, W. C., Yoshiyama, M., Ramage, A. G. *et al.* (1999). Modulation of voiding and storage reflexes by activation of alpha1-adrenoceptors. *European Urology* **36** (suppl 1), 68–73.

DeLancey, J. O. (1986). Correlative study of paraurethral anatomy. *Obstetrics and Gynecology* **68**, 91–97.

DeLancey, J. O. (1994). The anatomy of the pelvic floor. *Current Opinion in Obstetrics and Gynecology* **6**, 313–316.

DeLancey, J. O. (1996). Stress urinary incontinence: where are we now, where should we go? *American Journal of Obstetrics and Gynecology* **175**, 311–319.

Enhörning, G. (1961). Simultaneous recording of intravesical and intraurethral pressure: a study on urethral closure in normal and stress incontinent women. *Acta Chirurgica Scandinavica, Supplementum* **276**, 1–68.

Heesakkers, J. P. & Gerretsen, R. R. (2004). Urinary incontinence: sphincter functioning from a urological perspective. *Digestion* **69**, 93–101.

Kamo, I., Torimoto, K., Chancellor, M. B. *et al.* (2003). Urethral closure mechanisms under sneeze-induced stress condition in rats: a new animal model for evaluation of stress urinary incontinence. *American Journal of Physiology. Regulatory, Integrative and Comparative Physiology* **285**, R356–R365.

Kelly, H. & Dumm, W. (1914). Urinary incontinence in women, without manifest injury to the bladder. *Surgical Gynecology and Obstetrics* **18**, 444–453.

Kennedy, W. (1937). Incontinence of urine in the female, the urethral sphincter mechanism, damage of function, and restoration of control. *American Journal of Obstetrics and Gynecology* **34**, 576–589.

Kerns, J. M., Damaser, M. S., Kane, J. M. *et al.* (2000). Effects of pudendal nerve injury in the female rat. *Neurourology and Urodynamics* **19**, 53–69.

Kihara, K. & de Groat, W. C. (1997). Sympathetic efferent pathways projecting to the bladder neck and proximal urethra in the rat. *Journal of Autonomic Nervous System* **62**, 134–142.

Lose, G. (2001). Urethral pressure measurements. In *Textbook of Female Urology and Urogynaecology* (ed. L. Cardozo & D. Staskin), pp. 216–226. London: Health Publications.

Lose, G. & Colstrup. H. (1991). Urethral pressure and power generation during coughing and voluntary contraction of the pelvic floor in healthy females. *British Journal of Urology* **67**, 573–579.

Park, J. M., Bloom, D. A. & McGuire, E. J. (1997). The guarding reflex revisited. *British Journal of Urology* **80**, 940–945.

Petros, P. E. & Ulmsten, U. I. (1990). An integral theory of female urinary incontinence. Experimental and clinical considerations. *Acta Obstetrica et Gynecologica Scandinavica. Supplement* **153**, 7–31.

Slack, M., Tracey, M., Culligan, P. *et al.* (2004). Urethral retro-resistance pressure: a new clinical measure of urethral function. *Neurourology and Urodynamics* **23**, 656–661.

Smith, A. R, Hosker, G. L. & Warrell, D. W. (1989). The role of pudendal nerve damage in the aetiology of genuine stress incontinence in women. *British Journal of Obstetrics and Gynaecology* **96**, 29–32.

Snooks, S. J., Badenoch, D. F., Tiptaft, R. C. *et al.* (1985). Perineal nerve damage in genuine stress urinary incontinence. An electrophysiological study. *British Journal of Urology* **57**, 422–426.

Stevens, W. E. & Smith, S. (1937). Roentgenological examination of the female urethra. *Journal of Urology* **37**, 194–201.

Thind, P. & Lose G. (1994). The effect of bilateral pudendal blockade on the adjunctive urethral closure forces in healthy females. *Scandinavian Journal of Urology and Nephrology* **28**, 249–255.

Chapter 4

The social disability of stress urinary incontinence and the impact on service use and treatment patterns

Chris Shaw

It is accepted that stress urinary incontinence (SUI) can result in considerable social disability and quality of life impacts, although reports of the prevalence of disability are inconsistent due to variation in study methodology, such as differences in sample characteristics, measurement tools and definitions. Estimates range from less than 2% to 44% of women reporting socially disabling incontinence (McGrother 2003). It is generally agreed that such quality of life impacts increase with increasing severity of the condition (McGrother *et al.* 2004; Samuelsson *et al.* 1997). This is not, however, a perfect relationship and women can have relatively mild symptoms with considerable impact and vice versa, depending on their personal circumstances. For this reason, it is important to consider quality of life impacts when considering treatment options and also when assessing the outcome of interventions. In addition, incontinence is not a life threatening condition, but a troublesome condition for which improvement in quality of life may be a primary aim, particularly as complete cure is not always achieved or necessarily expected. Therefore, it is important to consider patient goals in relation to quality of life improvements as a major objective of treatment, or at the very least as a key addition to clinical measures of symptom improvement.

The degree of social disability experienced by women with SUI is integral to their help-seeking decisions and their motivation to carry out treatment procedures. It is, therefore, an essential component in the assessment of need and service planning. But the concept of quality of life and social disability is complex and research assessing quality of life is open to a wide range of interpretation. The aim of this chapter is to explore the relationship of social disability and quality of life impairments to women's illness behaviours and to health care professionals' treatment decisions, as well as presenting an overall view of the level of social disability resulting from SUI in the population.

Measurement of social disability

In outcome assessment and epidemiological studies, quantitative measures in the form of standardised questionnaires have been developed to measure quality of life and disability (Naughton *et al.* 2004). Generic measures assess broad concepts of quality of life that are useful in a research setting where comparison across patient groups and conditions is desirable but, because of their broad focus, they lack sensitivity. Condition-specific measures address those aspects of quality of life that are most likely to be affected by the condition under consideration. In relation to urinary incontinence, the impact of symptoms on social activities, relationships and feelings are those most frequently considered (Shaw *et al.* 2004a; Shumaker *et al.* 1994). In addition, several questionnaires address the bothersomeness of symptoms, either in general or in relation to individual symptoms (Naughton *et al.* 2004). Women frequently adopt management strategies that allow them to perform their daily activities, but these can involve considerable planning, effort, and inconvenience (Miteness 1987). The concept of bothersomeness taps into this impact on their lives where questions concerning limitations of activities may not.

Extent of social disability

The following data on the prevalence of social disability related to urinary incontinence comes from a survey done as part of the Leicestershire MRC Incontinence Study. 30,228 men and women, over the age of 40 years, who were community dwelling, resident in Leicestershire, and registered with a collaborating GP, were randomly selected to receive a mailed questionnaire. A response rate of 57.5% was achieved following two reminders. The survey contained questions concerning urinary symptoms of incontinence, frequency, urgency, and nocturia, impact on quality of life, service use in relation to urinary symptoms, general health and some demographic questions.

Social disability was defined as a response of 'a lot' to any one of the following questions: Do your urinary symptoms interfere with daily activities, social life, relationships or sleep, or upset/distress you, cause you physical discomfort, or affect your overall quality of life? (Response categories were 'a lot', 'a little' or 'not at all'.) The amount of 'bother' was also measured by the responses to two questions: "How much of a problem would you say you have with your urinary symptoms?" and "Do your urinary symptoms bother you?" Bothersome symptoms were defined by a response of 'severe' or 'moderate' to the first question or a response of 'a lot' to the second.

In total, 2303 (25%) women and 618 (7.7%) men reported experiencing clinically significant incontinence, defined as leakage several times a month or more often. 717 (7.7%) women reported stress incontinence symptoms only and 543 (5.8%) urge incontinence only (UUI), while 1043 (11.2%) had mixed symptoms of both stress and urge (MUI). In contrast, 42 (0.5%) men had SUI, 442 (5.5%) UUI and 134 (1.7%) MUI, showing the higher prevalence of incontinence in women. The majority of incontinent women experienced SUI either alone or in conjunction with urge symptoms. SUI is, therefore, a significant health concern in women over the age of 40 years living in the community, with nearly one in five women experiencing clinically significant SUI.

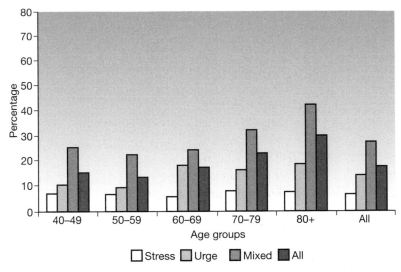

Figure 4.1 Social disablity by age and type of incontinence in women

Figure 4.1 shows the extent of disability in women by age and type of incontinence. Overall, 17.6% of women reported a lot of social disability resulting from urinary incontinence. This was greatest in those with MUI compared to those with isolated stress or urge symptoms. 6.7% of women with SUI experienced substantial impact on their social lives, and 14.1% of women with UUI. Overall, disabling incontinence was associated with increasing age, but this is not so clear cut when examining the different types of incontinence. Those with MUI show an age relationship, those with UUI to a lesser extent, and women with SUI have similar levels of disability across the age range.

Although most women did not report social disability, there were many more women who were bothered by symptoms: 40.8% of women with incontinence were bothered 'a lot' by their symptoms or found them a 'severe' or 'moderate' problem. Again, there is an overall relationship with increasing age and for each of the different types of incontinence, apart from SUI. Between 17% and 26% of women with SUI in each of the age groups were bothered by symptoms with a mean of 18% for all age groups (Figure 4.2).

Both disability and bothersomeness vary by the severity of leakage (measured as the amount of urine lost, with response categories of soaked, wet, damp, or almost dry) as can be seen in figures 4.3 and 4.4. Over 90% of women who are soaked and nearly 70% of women who are wet, experience symptoms as bothersome. Disability is also high in women who report severe leakage of 'soaked' or 'wet' with around 60% and 30% having 'a lot' of social disability respectively.

Although these data point to increasing age as a factor related to quality of life impairments, the relationship with severity suggests that the age effect may be

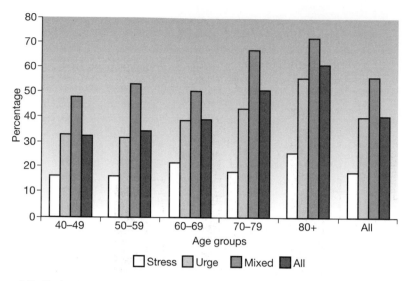

Figure 4.2 Bothersomeness by age and type of incontinence in women

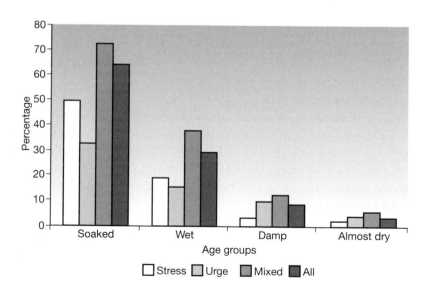

Figure 4.3 Disabling incontinence by severity in women

Table 4.1 Logistic regression analysis of predictors of social disability and bothersomeness.

Predictors	Odds ratio (confidence interval)	
Severity	**Bother**	**Disabling**
Soaked	42 (16,112)	29 (14,61)
Wet	11 (7,15)	8 (4,13)
Damp	3 (2,4)	2 (1,3)
Type of incontinence		
Urge	2 (2,3)	2 (1,3)
Mixed	4 (3,5)	3 (2,5)
Age		
50–59	ns	ns
60–69	ns	ns
70–79	1.4 (1,2)	ns
80+	2 (1,3)	ns

1998) (urge incontinent) of incontinent women. However, estimates over 50% tend to be based on selective samples of volunteers to advertisements rather than random population samples (Brown *et al.* 1998; Sandvik *et al.* 1993). Randomly selected samples of women covering the whole adult age range report estimates in the region of 35% (Simeonova & Bengtsson 1990), 13% (McGrother *et al.* 2004), or around 25% (Hannesad *et al.* 2002; Hunskaar *et al.* 2004). Studies focusing on older women sometimes give slightly higher estimates (Rekers *et al.* 1992) in line with other studies that report an age relationship, with older women more likely to seek help (Button *et al.* 1998). However, age effects may be confounded by duration and severity of symptoms as a relationship between help-seeking and severity is frequently reported (Button *et al.* 1998; Kinchen *et al.* 2002; Rekers *et al.* 1992). These figures also relate to all incontinence rather than stress incontinence. Help-seeking in women with SUI tends to be lower than in women with urge or mixed symptoms with around 15% of women with SUI seeking help and 32% and 34% of women with UUI and MUI seeking help (Shaw *et al.* 2004b). Figure 4.5 shows the prevalence of help-seeking in women with SUI found in the Leicester study. Overall 15.2% of women with SUI had sought help during the preceding 12 months. More women over the age of 60 years had sought help than younger women. In this sample, duration of symptoms was not associated with age although severity was (in terms of frequency of leakage but not amount of leakage), which may explain some of the age effect in help-seeking as older women experienced more frequent leakage. Figure 4.6 shows the relationship of help-seeking to quality of life impairments. 59% of those

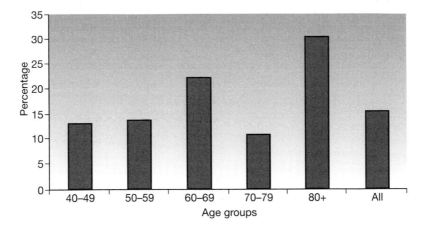

Figure 4.5 Help-seeking by age group in women with incontinence

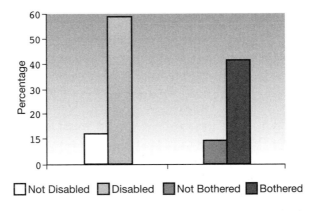

Figure 4.6 Percentage of women socially disabled or bothered by symptoms who have sought help

who report disabling symptoms had sought help compared with 12.7% of those not having disabling symptoms. Of those who were bothered by symptoms, 41.7% had sought help whereas only 9.9% of those who were not bothered sought help. A logistic regression analysis of the predictors of help-seeking which included age group, severity, disability, and bothersomeness found the quality of life variables to be the strongest predictors of help seeking with odds ratios and 95% confidence intervals of 3.8 (1.7, 8.6) and 4.1 (2.3, 7.1) for disability and bothersomeness respectively (Table 4.2). Severity of leakage was not independently associated with help-seeking in this

Table 4.2 Multivariate analysis of the predictors of help-seeking behaviour in women with incontinence.

Predictors	Odds Ratio (95% Confidence Interval)
Severity	
Soaked	3 (1,6)
Wet	ns
Damp	ns
Almost Dry	1
Type of incontinence	
Urge	ns
Mixed	1.4 (1,2)
Stress	1
Age (years)	
40–49	1
50–59	ns
60–69	ns
70–79	1.5 (1,2)
80+	3 (2,4)
Quality of life	
Disabling incontinence	3 (2,4)
Bothersome incontinence	3 (2,4)

analysis whereas age was, with those in the age groups 60–69 years and 80+ years, being twice as likely and 3.4 times more likely to seek help than those aged 40–49 years.

The data above show that although quality of life impairments are strong predictors of help-seeking more than half of the women who report having social disability or are bothered by their symptoms are not accessing services. Why are these women not expressing a need for services? A widely held view is that this is the hidden problem of incontinence and that there is a substantial level of unmet need in the general population. 'Embarrassment and stigma' is frequently considered to be one of the main reasons for failure to seek help, but this is just one of several reasons (Hagglund *et al.* 2003; Shaw *et al.* 2001). Other reasons which are often cited, that are borne out by research findings, are that symptoms are considered a normal part of female aging or an expected sequela of childbirth (Shaw *et al.* 2001; Simeonova & Bengtsson 1990). However, women with urinary symptoms also report the belief that no treatment is available or that they have low expectations of treatment (Rekers *et al.*

1992; Reymert & Hunskaar 1994). It is not surprising that women who hold such views do not seek help. But it is surprising and unfortunate that health care professionals sometimes reinforce these types of misattributions of cause and treatment of urinary symptoms (Shaw *et al*. 2001).

For women who believe that there is no treatment available for their symptoms there is no alternative but to develop strategies to cope with the condition from both a practical and psychological perspective. In adapting to living with symptoms a process of 'response shift' may take place in perceptions of quality of life (Ahmed *et al*. 2004). The concept of response shift has evolved from findings that people with illness and disability often have quality of life scores equivalent to those of healthy populations. It is also a common finding that people with deteriorating conditions adjust their perceptions and expectations to maintain a consistent quality of life (Ahmed *et al*. 2004). For example, if sport is a substantial aspect of an individual's life, and individuals find that they are no longer able to take an active part in their sport, they may focus their attention on training others or watching sports thus maintaining their basic interest but refocusing their expectations. This may explain why some women appear to have relatively little impairment in quality of life in the presence of severe symptoms, as they adapt their lifestyle to accommodate the symptoms. Deterioration in symptoms is often slow and adaptation of lifestyle a gradual process, and so the extent of adaptation is not always acknowledged. There may also, of course, be other factors influencing this finding, such as variations in personality characteristics, coping predispositions, and social circumstances, but the mismatch between the experience of quality of life, symptoms, and health behaviour warrants further research if we are to ensure equity of service provision, as explanations for non-access that involve low levels of awareness or education are likely to be most prominent in those who are also deprived in other ways.

A more simplistic explanation for the low levels of help-seeking is that some women acquire more effective coping strategies than others, thus preventing impact on their social lives. However, examination of the self care strategies reported by women in a subgroup of the Leicester UK sample suggest that the majority of strategies are avoidant in nature and unlikely to be effective in the longer term, particularly if symptoms deteriorate (Table 4.3). Similar findings have been reported in the literature (Herzog *et al*. 1989; Sandvik *et al*. 1993). This is in line with positive associations reported in some studies between duration of symptoms and help-seeking behaviour (Sandvik *et al*. 1993). There is limited evidence concerning the natural history of incontinence, but the epidemiology demonstrates a peak in prevalence of SUI at around 50 years of age with lower levels in older age. For some women the symptoms may remit and their coping strategies may be sufficient for their needs. But, in older age there is a rise in mixed and urge symptoms and maladaptive coping strategies developed in earlier life in relation to SUI, could lead to increasing levels of isolation and disability in those who develop more extensive problems in older age. This again, points to the importance of raising awareness in women and

Table 4.3 Management strategies reported by a subsample of responders in the Leicester study.

Management strategy	% of cases
Go to the toilet frequently	39.2
Use Pads/carry spare pads	22.7
Use other aids/keep aids close by	1.6
Go to the toilet before leaving the house	91.7
Only go to places where you know the location of toilet	14.3
Check for toilets on arriving somewhere	38.0
Avoid going out or particular situations	6.4
Restrict fluids	29.2
Take special diet	0 .5
Seek help from a health care professional	7.2
Talk to family/friends	6.7
Wear particular type of clothing	2.8
Use perfumes/deodorants	3.2
Sit on or stand at toilet a long time	20.5
Do exercises	18.8
Take medicine	5.0
Find information from books and leaflets	7.3
Other	2.9
1,636 valid cases	

providing information on the most effective ways to maintain urinary tract health and managing any problems that arise.

Patterns of treatment provision for SUI

There is little systematic information in the literature concerning patterns of treatment provision in primary care and while studies suggest that there is inconsistency there is insufficient information to assess quality. A study by Simeonova and Bengtsson (Simeonova & Bengtsson 1990) reported that 48% of the sample were told that UI is a common phenomenon which increases with age and that nothing can be done about it. 56% were referred for additional examination and 19% received no help. Goldstein *et al.* (Goldstein *et al.* 1992) found that 15% of women were referred to an urologist, 15% were advised to perform pelvic floor exercises, 10% were prescribed medication, 10% were advised to drink more fluids, 10% were told to return for a 6 month check, 5% to use protective pads and 30% were told that nothing could be done. Table 4.4 shows more recent data on treatment provision collected as part of the Leicester study.

Table 4.4 Treatment provided in those seeking help from a health care professional

Treatment	N (%)
Pelvic floor exercises	44 (40.4)
Bladder training	14 (12.8)
Referral to hospital	19 (17.4)
Antibiotics	27 (24.8)
Other medication	12 (11.0)
Reassurance	21 (19.3)
Told to return if symptoms get worse	38 (34.9)

40.4% of women with SUI were advised to carry out pelvic floor exercises, 17.4% were referred to hospital and 12.8% were advised on bladder training. Over one third were told to return if symptoms got worse. 4% of all the women with SUI reported having had surgery, the majority of these having had surgery more than 5 years previously. Overall 75% received some form of active treatment advice (pelvic floor exercises, referral to secondary care, bladder training, medication, or reassurance). Whether treatment was given or not was not related to frequency of leakage, social disability, or bother of symptoms in a logistic regression analysis. The only variable that was predictive of treatment was age, with younger women more likely to receive treatment than older women. These data suggest that although social disability and quality of life impacts are the main triggers for seeking help, they are not the key variables driving treatment decisions.

Another recent study that has examined treatment provision in women with SUI found that 23% received advice to carry out pelvic floor exercises, 57% received medication, 14% referred to hospital, 11% received dietary advice, 64% received reassurance, and just 6% were referred to a specialist nurse (Shaw et al. in press). What is striking about all these studies is that relatively few women are receiving pelvic floor therapy, which is the recommended first line treatment for SUI (Wilson et al. 2005), and few are accessing specialist continence nurses. Although newer treatments, such as duloxetine medication, are now available for women with SUI, the manufacturers recommend that it be given in conjunction with pelvic floor therapy for best effect and so it is important to continue to encourage behavioural treatments as well as appropriate lifestyle advice in order to ensure both short and longer term benefits.

Conclusions

Quality of life is an important aspect of the experience of women with incontinence and is also an important aspect of access to services and treatment provision. It is clear that help-seeking is not determined by symptoms alone, but on a complex set of factors which include symptom impact, coping resources, personal circumstances, awareness of the condition and treatment options, and attributions of causality. There is a need to improve patient knowledge and awareness to empower individuals to make appropriate health care choices and enable them to self manage symptoms in a more adaptive and effective way.

For those who choose medical help, symptom severity alone is not a sufficient indicator of treatment decisions or an adequate outcome indicator of treatment interventions. Treatment provision should focus more on patient goals in relation to their lifestyle aspirations. Education for health professionals who are first line contacts for women with incontinence is also required if we are to avoid reinforcing negative attitudes to incontinence and its treatment.

References

Ahmed, S., Mayo, N. E., Wood-Cauphinee, S., Hanley, J. A. & Cohen, S. R. (2004). Response shift influenced estimates of change in health-related quality of life post-stroke. *Journal of Clinical Epidemiology* **57**, 561–570.

Brown, J.S., Subak, L. L., Gras, J., Brown, B. A., Kuppermann, M. & Posner, S. F. (1998). Urge incontinence: the patient's perspective. *Journal of Women's Health* **7**, 1263–1269.

Button, D., Roe, B., Webb, C., Frith, T., Colin-Thorne, D. & Gardner, D. L. (1998). Consensus guidelines for the promotion and management of continence by primary health care teams: development, implementation and evaluation. *Journal of Advanced Nursing* **27**, 91–99.

Goldstein, M., Hawthorne, M. E., Engeberg, S., McDowell, B. J. & Burgio, K. L. (1992). Urinary incontinence: why people do not seek help. *Journal of Gerontological Nursing* **18**(4), 15–20.

Hagglund, D., Walker-Engstom, M.-L., Larsson, G. & Leppert, J. (2003). Reasons why women with long term urinary incontinence do not seek professional help: a cross-sectional population-based cohort study. *International Urogynecology Journal* **14**, 296–304.

Hannestad, Y. S., Rortveit, G. & Hunskaar, S. (2002). Help-seeking and associated factors in female urinary incontinence. The Norwegian EPINCONT Study. Epidemiology of Incontinence in the County of Nord-Trondelag. *Scandinavian Journal of Primary Health Care* **20**, 102–107.

Herzog, A. R., Fultz, N.H., Normolle, D.P., Brock, B. M. & Diokono, A. C. (1989). Methods used to manage urinary incontinence by older adults in the community. *Journal of the American Geriatric Society* **37**, 339–347.

Hunskaar, S., Lose, G., Sykes, D. & Voss S. (2004). The prevalence of urinary incontinence in women in four European countries. *British Journal of Urology International* **93**, 324–330.

Kinchen, K. S., Burgio, K., Diokno, A. C., Fultz, N. H., Bump, R. & Obenchain, R. (2002). Factors associated with women's decision to seek treatment for urinary incontinence. *Journal of Women's Health* **12**, 687–698.

McGrother, C. M. (2003). Urinary incontinence and storage symptoms: prevalence, impact and need for services in the UK 1960-2001. A systematic review. International continence Society 33rd Annual Meeting Florence, Italy, 5–9 October 2003.

McGrother, C. M, Donaldson, M. M. K., Shaw, C., Matthews, R. J., Hayward, T. A., Dallosso, H. M., Jagger, C., Clarke, M., Castleden, C. M. & the Leicestershire MRC Incontinence Study Team (2004). Storage symptoms of the bladder: prevalence, incidence and need for services in the UK. *British Journal of Urology International* **93**, 763–769.

Mitteness, L. S. (1987). So what do you expect when you're 85? Urinary incontinence in late life. *Research Social Health Care* **6**, 177–219.

Naughton, M. J., Donovan, J., Badia, X., Corcos, J., Gotoh, M., Kelleher, C., Lukacs, B. & Shaw, C. (2004). Symptom severity and QOL scales for urinary incontinence. *Gastroenterology,* **126,** 114–123.

Rekers, H., Drogendijk, A. C., Valkenburg, H. & Riphagen, F. (1992). Urinary incontinence in women from 35 to 79 years of age: prevalence and consequences. *Journal of Obstetrics Gynecology Reproductive Biology* **43**, 229–234.

Reymert, J. & Hunskaar, S. (1994). Why do only a minority of perimenopausal women with urinary incontinence consult a doctor? *Scandinavian Journal of Primary Health Care* **12**, 180–183.

Samuelsson, E., Victor, A. & Tibblin, G. (1997). A population study of urinary incontinence and nocturia among women aged 20–59 years. *Acta Ostetricia et Gynecologica Scandinavica* **76**, 74–80.

Sandvik, H., Kveine, E. & Hunskaar, S. (1993). Female urinary incontinence: psychosocial impact, self care, and consultations. *Scandinavian Journal Caring Science* **7**, 53–56.

Shaw, C., Brady, R., Allan, R., Jackson, C. & Hyde, C. (2001). Barriers to help-seeking in people with urinary problems. *Family Practice* **18**, 48–52.

Shaw, C., Matthews, R. J., Perry, S. I., Williams, K., Spiers, N., Assassa, R. P., McGrother, C., Dallosso, H., Jagger, C., Mayne. C. & Clarke, M. (2004a). Validity and reliability of a questionnaire to measure the impact of lower urinary tract symptoms on quality of life: The Leicester Impact scale. *Neurourology and Urodynamics* **23**, 229–236.

Shaw, C., DasGupta, R., Assassa, P. R., Martin, M., Abrams, P., Wagg, A., Mayne, C. & Bushnell, D. M. (2004b). The extent and severity of incontinence in a female primary care population. Society for Academic Primary Care Conference. Glasgow.

Shaw, C., Das Gupta, R., Bushnell, D. M,, Assassa, R. P., Abrams, P., Wagg, A., Mayne, C., Hardwick, C. & Martin, M. (in press). The extent and severity of urinary incontinence amongst women in UK GP waiting rooms. *Family Practice.*

Shumaker, S. A., Wyman, J. F., Uebersax, J. S., McClish, D., Fantl, J.A. for the continence Program in Women (CPW) Research Group (1994). Health-related quality of life measures for women with urinary incontinence: the Incontinence Impact Questionnaire and the Urogenital Distress Inventory. *Quality of Life Research* **3**, 291–306.

Simeonova, Z. & Bengtsson, C. (1990). Prevalence of urinary incontinence among women at a Swedish Primary Health Care Centre. *Scandinavian Journal of Primary Health Care* **8**, 203–206.

Wilson, P. D., Berghmans, B., Hagen, S., Hay Smith, J., Moore, K., Nygaard, I., Sinclair, L., Yamanishe, T. & Wyman, J. (2005). Adult Conservative Management. In *Incontinence. Third International Consultation on Incontinence*, vol. 2. (ed. Abrams, P., Cardozo, L., Khoury, S. & Wein, A.). Health Publication.

PART 2

Evidence and opinion for clinical assessment

Chapter 5

Evidence and opinion for medical assessment in primary care

Mike Kirby, Ann R. Wagg, Duncan S. Barron, David Stott and Kate Corlett

Urinary incontinence has been defined by the standardisation committee of the International Continence Society as 'the complaint of any involuntary leakage of urine' (Abrams *et al.* 2002, p. 3). The actual scale of the problem and its financial and social impact has only recently been appreciated. According to the Continence Foundation, one in four women and one in nine men will suffer from urinary incontinence at some stage of their lives (Norton 1994). It is a common problem at all ages, but is most prevalent in the elderly, especially among those living in institutions.

In the UK, there has been considerable progress raising public awareness of the effects of incontinence. Much work, in the form of publicity campaigns, has been done by the Continence Foundation, The Association for Continence Advice and *In*contact. Because of this, more patients are likely to request help for the problem. In a review of the literature Button *et al.* (1998) showed that help-seeking behaviour is increasingly common and could be due to development in health services and national campaigns for raising public awareness and education. Despite this publicity and the distribution of comprehensive guidelines on improving the detection and management of urinary incontinence, the problem remains common and undetected in older adults. This was highlighted in the National Service Framework for Older People (DH 2001).

Recent studies have shown that in the UK, over a 1 year period, over one-third of people aged 40 years plus (i.e. 9 million) are estimated to have a health care need for urinary storage symptoms, and one-fifth (i.e. 5 million) are estimated to require health care related to urinary symptoms, with unmet requirement affecting 3 million (McGrother *et al.* 2004). This represents a major public health problem. Furthermore, the costs of clinically significant urinary storage symptoms (CSUSS) in the community amounted to approximately 1.1% of overall NHS spending for 1999/2000. Intangible and personally borne costs are also important components of the cost of CSUSS. It also appears that there are large gender inequalities in the proportion of costs borne by the NHS, i.e. 91% of male NHS incontinence costs compared with 57% of female NHS incontinence costs (Turner *et al.* 2004). Despite a higher prevalence in women, men tend to make more general practitioner (GP) visits concerning incontinence problems resulting in more prescriptions and in-patient care.

In 2000, the NHS Review Group on Continence Services was convened which resulted in the publication of 'Good Practice in Continence Services' (Good Practice, DH 2000). This publication sets out to improve health and tackle inequalities in service provision for people with bowel and bladder dysfunction by outlining a standard set of principles. In an effort to deliver effective continence care, the document calls for new partnerships and different ways of working and sets out a proposal for an Integrated Continence Service (ICS) based on four levels of service provision:

- Level 1. Primary care
- Level 2. Specialist continence care
- Level 3. Consultant medical and surgical specialists
- Level 4. Regional or national centres of excellence

The proposal guidelines set out that primary and community health care teams should identify people with incontinence, offer appropriate assessments and help them and their carers understand the condition and offer any necessary treatment. The 'Good Practice' document also recommends that every primary health care team should: (1) have someone who is trained to undertake an informed continence assessment; (2) be in a position to facilitate access to specialist services when required; (3) carry out audits and; (4) complete the audit cycle.

'Good Practice' was published originally as a statement of best practice and therefore, does not prescribe mandatory actions for healthcare providers. However, it does set out in detail what is required for continence services at each level of the NHS and recommends evidence-based policies, procedures, guidelines and targets for the establishment of an integrated continence service (ICS). 'Good Practice' targets four areas for modernisation within continence services:

- Tools to improve service delivery
- Service organisation
- Service delivery
- Service commissioning

It has also helped establish milestones for the implementation of these recommendations, as defined in the Department of Health's National Service Framework for Older People (2001):

- April 2003: The development of an ICS by Health Improvement Programmes (HIMPs) and other relevant local plans.
- April 2004: An ICS should be established within all local health and social care systems.

- April 2005: Compliance with the Single Assessment Process (SAP) for each patient.

Education

A major obstacle in the improved management of urinary incontinence within primary care has been the lack of adequate training. A previous study indicated that there was a general lack of knowledge among GPs in the UK regarding the different types of incontinence (i.e. stress, urge and mixed: Brocklehurst 1990). A survey in Hertfordshire of 129 GPs in 1998 showed that 26% had no previous training in incontinence, 38% felt their training was inadequate and 67% felt guidelines would be helpful (Kirby 2004).

Definition

Incontinence is the main indicator of a storage disorder, which Abrams *et al.* (2002) define as: 'symptoms experienced during the storage phase of the bladder' (Abrams *et al.* 2002) and includes urgency, frequency and nocturia, as well as any leakage. Stress urinary incontinence (SUI) is involuntary leakage during, for example, effort, exertion, sneezing or coughing and is a common disorder among women of all ages, which compromises their quality of life (QoL) (Abrams *et al.* 2002).

SUI is the commonest of UI affecting women. The symptom of urge UI (UUI) is the complaint of involuntary leakage accompanied, or immediately preceded, by urgency (Abrams *et al.* 2002). Mixed UI (MUI) is a combination of both SUI and UUI. The problem for the physician or nurse is in determining the predominant symptoms and therefore what treatments are most likely to help.

Causes

To manage stress incontinence effectively it is helpful to have an understanding of the underlying cause(s). SUI is thought to occur because of bladder neck/urethral hypermobility and/or neuromuscular defects in the intrinsic sphincter (Koelbl *et al.* 2002). The result is that urine leaks whenever the urethral resistance is exceeded by an increase in intra-abdominal pressure.

Impact

Problems with personal hygiene may lead to the avoidance of sexual relationships and leakage restricts physical activity (Fultz *et al.* 2003). Surprisingly, less than 40% of women with urinary incontinence (UI) seek appropriate medical attention (Kinchen *et al.* 2003; Hunskaar *et al.* 2004). Many women are too embarrassed to talk about the problem and it is often considered a normal part of aging (Fultz *et al.* 2003). Late presentation is also determined by lack of knowledge about possible treatments and a fear of surgical procedures.

Prevalence of urinary incontinence

Prevalence has been studied extensively among different target groups using various survey designs. A recent review of the worldwide prevalence of UI reveals that the median prevalence of female UI is 27.6% (Minassian *et al.* 2003). The prevalence rates of UI in institutional settings range from 6 to 72%, depending on the definition (Hunskaar *et al.* 2002). UI is about twice as prevalent among women as men (McGrother *et al.* 2003). Several large surveys have reported the relative proportions of SUI, MUI and UUI. The data show that pure SUI is the most frequently reported symptom of UI, accounting for about half the female patients. Pure UUI affects 10–20% of incontinent women and 30–40% have symptoms of MUI. Clearly, as MUI is a combination of SUI and UUI, most women, regardless of age, complain of SUI with or without additional lower urinary tract symptoms (LUTS).

The large Norwegian EPINCONT survey collected data from 27,936 women aged older than 20 years, living in one county in Norway between 1995 and 1997 (Hunskaar *et al.* 2000). Twenty-five per cent of women were found to have urinary leakage, with SUI being the most commonly reported disorder. SUI symptoms are thought to affect approximately one in three women over 18 years old in the UK (Hunskaar *et al.* 2004)

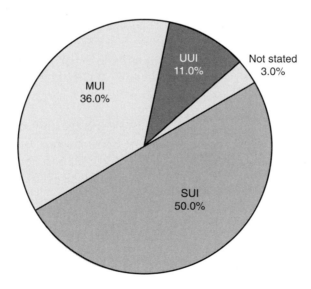

Figure 5.1 Predominance of SUI (Hannestad *et al.* 2000)

Risk factors and age distribution

Knowledge of risk factors allows for targeted case finding. Some risk factors for developing SUI include (Viktrup 2002):

- Weak collagen
- Age
- Childbirth
- Obesity
- Constipation
- Advanced pelvic organ prolapse
- Chronic obstructive airways disease

The EPINCONT study also confirmed the impact of age on the prevalence of UI and the fact that SUI is more common in younger and middle-aged women, whereas MUI predominantly occurs in older women (Hannestad *et al.* 2000).

The identification of sufferers and screening opportunities

'If doctors and nurses don't ask, patients don't tell'

New patient registrations, health promotion clinics and routine consultations are ideal situations in which to reinforce strategies which may detect and prevent incontinence. Such strategies include exercise regimes, weight control, healthy diet (especially to avoid constipation), treatment of chronic cough, the use of hormone replacement therapy in women and the assessment of prostatic disease in males. In the elderly, correction of impaired mobility to facilitate access to toilets and an adequate fluid intake to avoid dehydration, are important.

Medical management of LUTS caused by bladder outlet obstruction in men will reduce detrusor overactivity and consequent urge incontinence. But alpha-blockers (used for treating hypertension and LUTS) may relax the bladder neck and exacerbate stress incontinence in both men and women. Opportunities arise during routine consultations to assess not only those patients who complain of incontinence, but also those who do not present with any complaint. There may be obvious odour or wetness and specific targeted questions such as 'do you ever lose urine when you don't want to?' or 'do you wear a pad or other protection to soak up urine?', are more likely to result in a positive response than traditional inquiries such as 'how are your water works?'.

Regular review of older people is an ideal opportunity for assessing bladder function in an 'at risk' population. These checks may be performed by the practice nurse, district nurse or health visitor and this may well be done in the patient's home. Identifying patients in this manner may well reduce the likelihood of premature admission to residential or nursing care (Thom *et al.* 1997).

Opportunities to identify patients suffering from bladder problems in general practice occur in day-to-day practice. Examples of this are (Cardozo *et al.* 2001, p. 38):

- Nursing and residential homes
- Well woman and well man clinics
- New patient medicals/questionnaires
- Over 75 year old checks
- Postnatal examinations
- Cervical smear clinics
- Family planning clinics
- Posters and literature in waiting rooms

Assessment

The assessment of patients with bladder problems is ideally done in the primary care setting. Thakar and Stanton (2000) assert that in caring for women with UI there should be an emphasis on primary care assessment and management, as it provides both short and long term benefits. This approach benefits secondary care by ensuring that only patients who cannot be satisfactorily managed in primary care are referred. It may also benefit the patient with simple UI who may not need to undergo uncomfortable assessment such as urodynamics. Thus, efficiency in the referral process may benefit both the quality and cost of care.

There is general agreement in the many national guidelines regarding the initial history and symptom assessment of UI in women (Viktrup *et al.* 2004). The International Consultation on Incontinence (ICI) guideline differentiates between simple and complex cases (Abrams *et al.* 2000 p. 2156). In the interests of patient safety, in the initial assessment there is a need to distinguish women with relatively simple presentations of UI from those with more complex cases requiring specialist evaluation earlier in the course of their urinary dysfunction. The guidelines suggest that there are three main symptom categories that should be considered during the initial assessment of women with no complex history (SUI, UUI and MUI). A complex history includes any of the following:

- Recurrent incontinence
- Incontinence symptoms accompanied by pain
- Haematuria
- Recurrent infection
- Voiding symptoms
- History of pelvic irradiation
- Radical pelvic surgery
- Women who present with a significant post-void residual urine volume (PVR)
- Advanced pelvic organ prolapse
- Suspected malignancy

Such cases should be more carefully evaluated and referred for management in secondary care (Abrams *et al.* 2000).

Abrams *et al.*'s (2002) guidelines detail the initial management of urinary incontinence in women and is useful in both the primary and secondary care setting. At the current time, much progress needs to be made. History taking by the primary health care team can be time consuming, examination may be embarrassing and for many primary care physicians, the temptation to refer to a specialist may be overwhelming. As highlighted earlier, inadequate training has been a major obstacle to the improved management of urinary incontinence in primary care. This was

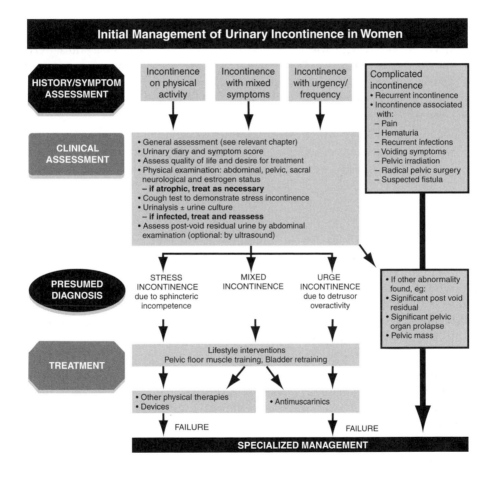

Figure 5.2 Initial management of urinary incontinence (Abrams *et al.* 2002; European Association of Urology Guidelines 1999 in Viktrup *et al.* 2004)

confirmed fifteen years ago in two studies, which demonstrated a lack of knowledge among general practitioners regarding the treatment of the types of incontinence and their causes, assessment and evaluation (Brocklehurst 1990, 1993).

The initial approach to diagnosing all bladder problems is a detailed medical history and thorough physical examination of the patient. This can be satisfactorily done in primary care either by the GP, or a practice nurse with the relevant expertise. There is no reason why this cannot be a comprehensive assessment as detailed in the ICI guideline. An accurate diagnosis should be made and a trial of appropriate treatment initiated (O'Brien & Long 1995). Patients who have a complex history should be referred to secondary care. A recommended approach to the diagnosis of bladder problems includes:

- Taking important aspects of the medical history include: e.g. history, pattern and extent of the urinary problems and any associated symptoms. A relatively short and focused history will distinguish SUI from UUI (Table 5.1).
- The mobility of the patient and environmental factors, mental state, medical and surgical history focusing on abdominal and pelvic surgery.
- Obstetric history
- Fluid intake and diet
- Medication history (see below)

Medication history

Drugs and other substances that might be implicated in urinary symptoms include (Cardozo *et al.* 2001, p.33):

- Diuretics
- Antidepressants
- Calcium channel blockers
- Antihistamines
- Benzodiazepines/sedatives/hypnotics
- Phenothiazines
- Alpha blockers
- Atropinic inhalers
- Alcohol
- Caffeine

The physical examination should cover the following aspects:

- The abdomen to detect masses, suprapubic fullness or tenderness and, if possible, a post-void residual urine estimation.
- Examination of the perineal area to assess the condition of the skin, look for soreness or wetness and check for genital atrophy, prolapse and pelvic mass.

Table 5.1 Useful questions to aid diagnosis of urinary symptoms (Cardozo *et al.* 2001)

Question	Symptoms	Overactive bladder	Stress incontinence	Mixed incontinence
How often do you go to the toilet during the day?	Frequency (>7 micturations/ 24 hour period)	Yes	Sometimes	No
Do you wake up more than once at night needing to go to the toilet?	Nocturia	Usually	Seldom	Usually
Do you ever have to hurry to reach the toilet in time?	Urgency	Yes	No	Yes
Do you ever *not* reach the toilet in time?	Urge incontinence	Often	No	Often
Do you ever leak urine when you laugh, sneeze, cough, jump or run?	Stress incontinence	No	Always	Always
If you leak, is it just a little drop or is it sometimes quite a lot more?	Amount of leakage (if present	Large (usually)	Small	Large
		Treat as overactive bladder	Treat as stress incontinence	Treat predominant symptoms

- Assess the pelvic floor tone.
- Examine carefully to exclude faecal impaction and vaginal foreign bodies.
- In men, in addition to abdominal examination, a digital rectal examination should be performed to assess the prostate gland. (Stress incontinence is rare in men unless they have had urological surgery or have neurological disease).
- In women a simple objective test for stress incontinence can be performed by asking the patient, (with a reasonably full bladder), to stand with legs apart so that the urethral orifice can be seen. She is then asked to cough and resulting leakage of urine demonstrates the problem. This can be embarrassing for the patient and a clear explanation of the reason for the test can be reassuring.

If clinically indicated, a general physical examination should be included, looking for oedema or neurological abnormality, especially of the S2–S4 segments. The patient's general mobility, manual dexterity and mental state should be assessed. A sample of urine should be sent for culture and sensitivities and, if there is haematuria, for cytology.

Other assessments that are helpful include a voiding record and environmental and social factors such as frailty and access to toilets, which can be contributory factors especially when there is urgency. When deemed clinically appropriate, blood tests can be performed to assess renal function, glucose and calcium. In those patients who have haematuria or irritative symptoms, urine cytology is essential and referral to an urologist should follow to exclude malignancy.

Early diagnosis and the treatment of incontinence to prevent ongoing problems is the key to success. The involvement of general practitioners, practice nurses and district nurses, in association with a community based specialist nurse and continence advisors, can avoid the delay caused by specialist referral.

Primary care teams should be managing patients with incontinence. Many studies have shown that conservative management in the community is highly efficacious. Conservative management includes bladder retraining programs for detrusor overactivity, which have shown success rates of up to 85%, while pelvic floor exercises for SUI are successful in 65% of cases (Hahn *et al.* 1993). It has been shown that improvements made in attending a nurse run clinic in primary care can be maintained for up to four years in 69% of patients (O'Brien & Long 1995; O'Brien 1996).

Symptom questionnaires

Questionnaires can be used to assess the prevalence of urinary symptoms and incontinence and the impact on a patient's quality of life. Such instruments may measure the severity of symptoms and have the advantage of being non-invasive, inexpensive and often self-administered. In practice, only a few such specific instruments assessing incontinence have been adequately validated, those that have include the King's Health Questionnaire (KHQ: Kelleher *et al.* 1997) and the Bristol Lower Urinary Tract Symptom Questionnaire (Jackson *et al.* 1996), both of which are discussed later. Other tools, for example the Nottingham Health Profile (NHP: Kind & Carr-Hill 1987), have been considered too generic in their approach. The NHP has 38 questions covering six broad health categories. Although a good indicator of general well-being, the authors argued that it had not proven to be sensitive enough for specific conditions such as incontinence, because none of the categories dealt with diagnostic data regarding urinary symptoms.

An example of a specific incontinence instrument includes one developed by Resnick *et al.* (1994), but this evaluated incontinence only and not other forms of lower urinary tract symptoms or effect on quality of life. Bo (1994) reported an instrument evaluating female stress incontinence and the effect on social activity. For this study, two instruments were designed. One was a leakage test listing thirteen situations where leakage might occur, the other being a social activity index listing nine activities that might be affected by the possibility of leakage. In a similar design, a Urological Distress Inventory and an Incontinence Impact Questionnaire have been used in combination by Shumaker *et al.* (1994) to determine the effect incontinence has on women. These instruments have been found to have good reliability and validity and are highly recommended (Naughton *et al.* 2004). Used in combination, these instruments gathered information on symptoms and effect on certain activities.

Jackson *et al.* (1996) reported the development of the Bristol Female Lower Urinary Tract Symptom Questionnaire. Although it was found to produce good psychometric validity and reliability, it comprised of several pages which, if used in a clinical setting, would impact on consultation time, an obvious problem in the primary care environment. However, Swithinbank *et al.* (1999) successfully used this questionnaire for a postal survey and achieved an 80% response rate. This suggests that given time at home, longer questionnaires can be useful. However, in primary care, in a clinical setting, time is limited.

The most widely used questionnaire assessing urinary incontinence in women has been developed at King's College Hospital and is known as the King's Health Questionnaire (KHQ: Kelleher *et al.* 1997). This is a disease-specific health related quality of life (HRQoL) instrument used to assess patients with urinary incontinence. It has been widely used in clinical studies as a valid, reliable and clinically sensitive endpoint (Homma *et al.* 2004). It includes 20 questions relating to symptoms of urinary incontinence. In a study involving 239 women referred for urinary investigations, the questionnaire was shown to be a valid instrument for the assessment of quality of life in women with urinary incontinence (Reese *et al.* 2003). Although shorter than the Bristol Female Lower Urinary Tract Symptoms Questionnaire, it is still several pages long. It is used in specialist clinics and in hospital practice where it is usually given to the patient to complete before seeing the consultant physician or nurse.

Use in primary care

Questionnaires need to be convenient and easy to understand and possess sufficiently good psychometric properties and sensitivity to clinical change. There are times when a short form of a HRQoL questionnaire is desired, for example when used for frequent assessment, or when the assessment time is very limited. In these situations, answering many questions is time-consuming and this may increase the number of unanswered items. Researchers often prefer to use shorter forms unless there is a specific and clear need for detail on certain symptoms. For this reason, the Incontinence Impact Questionnaire (IIQ: Shumaker *et al.* 1994) and the Urogenital Distress Inventory (UDI: Uebersax *et al.* 1995) have short-form versions.

The International Prostate Symptom Score (I-PSS: Barry *et al.* 1992) has been found suitable for use in the primary care setting with men. The IPSS was originally developed by the American Urological Association to evaluate the impact and severity of symptoms in men with benign prostatic hyperplasia (BPH) and it is still one of the main instruments used for this purpose (Barry *et al.* 1992). It is widely used in urological and primary care around the world for use in men with LUTS.

The IPSS questionnaire was originally administered to patients known to have BPH in order to assess the discriminative validity of the instrument. Cronbachs alpha and Pearson's correlation coefficients revealed that the tool was both reliable and valid. The instrument is easy to complete, comprising just eight questions, graded on a Likert-type scale of 1–5, to assess obstructive and irritative symptoms. Quality of life effects are assessed with a single question. It has also been used to evaluate voiding behaviour and its impact on quality of life in women (Desgrandchamps *et al.* 1996). Quality of life was reported to be positively correlated with irritative symptoms in women. The most troublesome voiding disorder was urgency.

The Female Urinary Symptom Score (FUSS: Wagg 2004) was adapted from the I-PSS to provide a short and easy to use questionnaire to assess urinary incontinence and lower urinary tract symptoms in women.

Two of the I-PSS questions dealing with intermittency and weak stream, which are predominantly male problems, were replaced with questions relating to stress incontinence and urge incontinence, these being two of the most commonly reported voiding disorders in the literature on women (Perry & Shaw 2000). The two symptoms relating to intermittency and weak stream are generally associated with obstruction. Desgrandchamps *et al.* (1996), who used the questionnaire unchanged for women, noted this and the lack of questions on incontinence. Question 3 in the IPSS ('over the past month or so how often have you found you stopped and started again several times when you urinated?'), was replaced with 'over the past month, how often have you lost urine on laughing, coughing or sneezing?'. IPSS question 5 ('over the past month or so how often have you had a weak urinary stream?'), was replaced with 'over the past month or so how often have you leaked urine before reaching the toilet?'.

In a study of elderly men to test the specificity of the I-PSS questionnaire, women were used as the control (Chai *et al.* 1993). Two groups were used: one selected from attendees at a urology clinic and the other group from the general population. It was found that while total scores were similar, women scored higher for frequency and urgency in the clinic group and the men scored higher for the obstructive symptoms. This supported the decision to modify the questionnaire for women. In order to validate the FUSS questionnaire, it was decided to use the KHQ as a comparator because of its wide use in multinational clinical studies and proven reliability and validity.

The FUSS questionnaire and the King's Health Questionnaire were sent to 220 women aged between 45 and 65 years randomly selected from two general practices in the UK. Total scores on each instrument were compared for each woman and correlated. Each woman was sent the FUSS questionnaire two weeks later to enable a re-test reliability score to be calculated.

Responses to both the FUSS and the King's Health Questionnaire were received from 158 (72%) of the 220 women. The FUSS questionnaire was generally completed more fully (94%), than the King's Health Questionnaire (73%). Correlation between total scores on both questionnaires was high at Pearson's $r = 0.83$, $n = 115$, $p < 0.001$. Individual correlation coefficients between similar items on both questionnaires varied from 0.56 (urgency) to 0.86 (stress incontinence). There was no single quality of life score in the King's Health Questionnaire, although several questions related to quality of life.

Response rate to the test-retest of the FUSS questionnaire was high. Of the 158 women who were sent the questionnaire a second time, 137 (87%) responded and of these 131 (96%) were filled in completely. The women were grouped according to score as mild (1–8), moderate (9–20) and severe (>20). At re-test, 103 of the 131 individuals (78.6%) were placed in the same category as on the first test. Moreover, all the 'transfers' were to the adjacent category. Thus, 91% (71/78) of those whose first test was classified as mild were allocated to mild on re-test and the remainder were allocated to 'moderate'. Similarly, all the individuals who were categorised as 'mild' at re-test were either mild (87.7%) or moderate (13.3%) at first test. There were no cases where an individual moved from mild to severe or vice-versa. The correlation between total scores at re-testing was high at $r = 0.88$, $n = 131$, $p < 0.001$.

The FUSS questionnaire has proved to be valid and reliable in a comparison with the KHQ. A prevalence study has subsequently been completed and an intervention study is underway using the questionnaire and will be reported later. It is hoped that the questionnaire can be used widely to provide a valid and simple way to assess LUTS in women and offer primary care professionals an opportunity, in the primary care setting, to provide them with appropriate investigation and treatment.

Management

The ICI guidelines recommend that the initial treatment of UI in women include lifestyle interventions in addition to therapies aimed as specific types of incontinence (Abrams *et al.* 2000). Similar to the ICI recommendations, The Royal College of Obstetricians and Gynaecologists (RCOG 2002) guidelines call for the initial treatment of presumed SUI, detrusor overactivity and combinations of the two with lifestyle interventions, pelvic floor muscle training (PFMT) and bladder retraining. The RCOG (2002) recommendations also advise considering adding antimuscarinic agents for patients with presumed detrusor overactivity and combinations of presumed detrusor overactivity and SUI in patients who do not improve with the above therapies (Royal College of Obstetricians and Gynaecologists 42nd Study Group 2002).

The advent of a new and effective treatment for SUI will undoubtedly lead to modification of the guidelines (ICI Guidelines 2002; Abrams *et al.* 2005). Duloxetine, a potent and balanced dual serotonin and noradrenaline reuptake inhibitor (SNRI), is developing an evidence base to fulfil this need (Norton *et al.* 2002).

Table 5.2 Female Urinary Symptom Score (FUSS) adapted from the International Prostate Symptom Score (Barry et al. 1992)

Patient Identification:　　　Date:

	Not at all	Less than 1 time in 5	Less than half the time	About half the time	More than half the time	Almost always	Fill in your score
1. Incomplete emptying Over the past month, how often have you had a sensation of not emptying your bladder completely after you finish urinating?	0	1	2	3	4	5	
2. Frequency Over the past month, how often have you had to urinate again less than two hours after you finished urinating?	0	1	2	3	4	5	
3. Stress incontinence Over the past month, how often have you lost urine on laughing, coughing, or sneezing?	0	1	2	3	4	5	
4. Urgency Over the past month, how often have you found it difficult to postpone urination?	0	1	2	3	4	5	
5. Urge incontinence Over the past month, how often have you leaked urine before reaching the toilet?	0	1	2	3	4	5	
6. Straining Over the past month, how often have you had to push or strain to begin urination?	0	1	2	3	4	5	

Table 5.2 Continued...

	None	1 Time	2 Times	3 Times	4 Times	5 times or more	Fill in your score
7. Nocturia Over the past month, how many times did you most typically get up to urinate from the time you went to bed at night until the time you got up in the morning?	0	1	2	3	4	5	
Total score							
Quality of Life due to Urinary Symptoms	Delighted	Pleased	Mostly Satisfied	Mixed	Mostly Dissatisfied	Unhappy	Terrible
If you were to spend the rest of your life with your urinary condition just the way it is now, how would you feel about that? *(Please circle appropriate number)*	0	1	2	3	4	5	6

Conclusion

Current guidelines put primary care in the forefront of the identification and management of urinary incontinence. Stress incontinence is a common disorder among women of all ages, which can compromise their quality of life.

Successful management, resulting in the relief of symptoms of incontinence, depends on an accurate and comprehensive assessment followed by appropriate advice and follow-up. Women and men need to be informed that help for many urinary complaints is available and that treatment is effective. Members of the primary health care team should be encouraged to elicit urinary complaints from females and males because if doctors and nurses do not ask, patients do not tell.

Education and training are essential as Primary Care Trusts move towards an Integrated Continence Service. The treatment and follow-up will be multidisciplinary, involving not only doctors and nurses, but also physiotherapists, occupational therapists and social workers.

All those of us working in primary care who deal with patients with urinary disorders need to be sensitive to the great emotional and social distress associated with these complaints and deal with them sensitively and sympathetically.

Acknowledgements

We thank Stephanie Cooper for her detailed and helpful comments on an earlier draft of this chapter.

References

Abrams, P., Lowry, S. K., Wein, A. J., Bump, R., *et al.* (2000). Assessment and treatment of urinary incontinence, *The Lancet* **355** 2153–2158.

Abrams, P., Cardozo, L. *et al.* (2002). The standardisation of terminology of lower urinary tract function: Report from the standardisation Sub-committee of the International Continence Society. *Neurourology and Urodynamics* **21**, 167–178.

Abrams, P., Cardozo, L., Khoury, S., Wen, A. (Eds). (2005). Incontinence. 3rd International Consultation on Incontinence. Public Health Publications Ltd. Monaco 2004.

Barry, M., Fowler, F. *et al.* (1992). The American Urological Association symptom index for benign prostatic hyperplasia. *Journal of Urology* **148**, 1549–1557.

Bo, K. (1994). Reproducibility of instruments designed to measure subjective evaluation of female stress urinary incontinence. *Scandinavian Journal of Urology and Nephrology* **28**, 97–100.

Brocklehurst, J. C. (1990). Professional and public education about incontinence. A British experience. *Journal of the American Geriatrics Society* **38**, 384–386.

Brocklehurst, J. C. (1993). Urinary incontinence in the community - analysis of a MORI poll. *British Medical Journal* **306**, 832–834.

Button, D., Roe, B., Webb, C. *et al.* (1998). *Continence: Promotion and Management by the Primary Health Care Team: Consensus Guidelines*. London: Whurr Publishers.

Chai, T., Belville, W., *et al.* (1993). Specificity of the American Urological Association voiding symptom index: Comparison of unselected and selected samples of both sexes. *Journal of Urology* **150**, 1710–1713.

Desgrandchamps, F., Cortesse, A. S. *et al.* (1996). Normal voiding behaviour in women. *European Urology* **30**, 18–23.

Department of Health (2001) *National Service Framework for Older People*, London: DH. Available online at: http://www.dh.gov.uk/assetRoot/04/07/12/83/04071283.pdf [Accessed 12 January 2005.]

Department of Health (2000): *Good Practice in Continence Services*. London: DH Available online at: http://www.dh.gov.uk/assetRoot/04/05/75/29/04057529.pdf [Accessed 12 January 2005.]

Fultz, N. H., Burgio, K. *et al.* (2003). Burden of stress urinary incontinence for community-dwelling women. *American Journal of Obstetrics and Gynecology* **189**, 1275–1282.

Hahn, I., Milson, I. *et al.* (1993). Long term results of pelvic floor training in female stress urinary incontinence. *British Journal of Urology* **72**, 421–427.

Hannestad, Y. S., Rortveit, G. *et al.* (2000). A community-based epidemiological survey of female urinary incontinence: The Norwegian Epincont Study. *Journal of Clinical Epidemiology* **53**: 1150–1157.

Homma, Y. & Uemura, S. (2004). Use of the short form of King's Health Questionnaire to measure quality of life in patients with an overactive bladder. *BJU International* **93**, 1009–1013.

Hunskaar, S., Arnold, E. P. *et al.* (2000). Epidemiology and natural history of urinary incontinence. *International Urogynecology Journal and Pelvic Floor Dysfunction* **11**, 301–319.

Hunskaar S, Burgio K *et al.* (2002). Epidemiology and natural history of urinary incontinence. In *Incontinence*, 2nd edn (ed. P. Abrams, L. Cardozo, *et al.*), pp, 165–201. Plymouth, UK: Health Publication Ltd.

Hunskaar, S., Lose, G. *et al.* (2004). Prevalence of urinary incontinence in women in four European countries. *BJU International* **93**, 324–330.

Jackson, S., Donovan, J. *et al.* (1996). The Bristol Female Lower Urinary Tract symptom questionnaire: development and psychometric testing. *British Journal of Urology* **77**, 805–812.

Kelleher, C., Cardozo, L. *et al.* (1997). A new questionnaire to assess the quality of life of urinary incontinent women. *British Journal of Obstetrics and Gynaecology* **104**, 1374–1379.

Kinchen, K. S., Burgio, K. *et al.* (2003). Factors associated with women's decisions to seek treatment for urinary incontinence. *Journal of Women's Health* **12**, 687–698.

Kind, P. & Carr-Hill, R. (1987). The Nottingham Health Profile: a useful tool for epidemiologists? *Social Science and Medicine* **25**, 905–910.

Kirby, M. (2004). Evidence and opinion for assessment in primary care. Paper given at the Key Advances in the Effective Management of Stress Urinary Incontinence [Inaugural] Annual Update, Royal College of Obstetricians and Gynaecologists, London, 17 December 2004.

Koelbl, H., Mostwin, J. *et al.* (2002). Pathophysiology. In *Incontinence*, 2nd edn (ed. P. Abrams, L. Cardozo *et al.*), pp.165–201. Plymouth, UK: Health Publication Ltd.

McGrother, C. W., Donaldson, M. M. K., Shaw, C. *et al.* (2004). Storage symptoms of the bladder: prevalence, incidence and need for services in the UK. *British Journal of Urology* **93**, 763–769.

McGrother, C. M., Donaldson, M., Wagg, A. *et al.* (2003). Continence. In: *Health Care Needs Assessment: The epidemiology based needs assessment reviews*, (ed. R. J. M. J. Stevens). Abingdon: Radcliffe Medical Press.

Minassian, V. A., Drutz, H. P. *et al.* (2003). Urinary incontinence as a worldwide problem. *International Journal of Gynaecology and Obstetrics* **82**, 327–338.

Naughton, M. J., Donovan, J., Badia X, Corcos J, Gotoh M, Kelleher C, Lukacs B, Shaw C. (2004). Symptom severity and QoL scales for urinary incontinence, *Gastroenterology* **126**, S114–S123.

Norton, C. (1994). Increasing incontinence awareness. *Journal of Community Nursing* **February**, 8–12.

Norton, P. A., Zinner, N. R. *et al.* (2002). Duloxetine versus placebo in the treatment of stress urinary incontinence. *American Journal of Obstetrics and Gynecology* **187**, 40–48.

O'Brien, J. (1996). Evaluating primary care interventions for incontinence. *Nursing Standard* **10**, 40–43.

O'Brien, J. & Long, H. (1995). Urinary incontinence: Long term effectiveness of nursing intervention in primary care. *British Medical Journal* **311**, 1208.

Perry, S. & Shaw, C. (2000). An epidemiological study to establish the prevalence of urinary symptoms and felt need in the community: The Leicestershire MRC Incontinence Study. *Journal of Public Health Medicine* **22**, 427–434.

Reese, P. R., Pleil, A. M., Okano, G. J. *et al.* (2003). Multinational study of reliability and validity of the King's Health Questionnaire in patients with overactive bladder. *Quality of Life Research* **12**, 427–442.

Resnick, N., Beckett, L. *et al.* (1994). Short term variability of Self Report of Incontinence in Older Persons. *Journal of the American Geriatrics Society* **42**, 202–207.

Royal College of Obstetricians and Gynaecologists 42nd Study Group (2002). Incontinence in women – study group recommendation. London: RCOG. Available online at http://www.rcog.org.uk/mainpages.asp?PageID=754. [Accessed 18 January 2005.]

Shaw, P. (2001). Evidence and opinion for medical assessment in the primary care setting. *The Effective Management of Detrusor Instability* (ed. L. Cardozo, C. Chapple, and A. Miles). pp. 29–39. London: Aesculapius Medical Press.

Shumaker, S., Wyman, J. *et al.* (1994). Health related QoL measures for women with urinary incontinence: The incontinence Impact questionnaire and the Urological Distress Inventory. Continence Programme in Women (CPM) Research Group. *Quality of Life Research* **3**, 291–306.

Swithinbank, L., Donovan, J. L. *et al.* (1999). Urinary symptoms and incontinence in women: relationships between occurrence, age and perceived impact. *British Journal of General Practice* **49**, 897–900.

Thakar, R. & Stanton, S. (2000). Management of urinary incontinence in women. *British Medical Journal* **321**, 1326–1331.

Thom, D. H. *et al.* (1997). Hospitalisation, nursing home admission and mortality. *Age and Aging* **26**, 367–374.

Turner, D. A., Shaw, C., McGrowther, C. W. *et al.* (2004). The cost of clinically significant urinary storage symptoms for community dwelling adults in the UK. *BJU International* **93**, 1246–1252.

Uebersax, J. S., Wyman, J. F., Shumaker, S. A. *et al.* (1995). Short forms to assess life quality and symptom distress for urinary incontinence in women: the Incontinence Impact Questionnaire and the Urogenital Distress Inventory. *Neurourology and Urodynamics* **14**, 131–139.

Viktrup, L. (2002). Female stress and urge incontinence in family practice: insight into the lower urinary tract. *International Journal of Clinical Practice* **56**, 694–700.

Viktrup, L., Summers, K. H. *et al.* (2004). Clinical practice guidelines for the initial management of urinary incontinence in women: a European-focused review. *BJU International* **94** (Suppl. 1), 14–22.

Wagg, A. R. (2004). A modified symptom score for female incontinence. Paper given at *The Royal College of Nursing Continence Care Conference*, York, UK, 3 and 4 November 2004.

Chapter 6

Evidence and opinion for advanced nursing assessment in secondary care

Kate Anders

Introduction

Stress urinary incontinence (SUI) is the complaint of involuntary leakage on effort or exertion, or on sneezing or coughing (Abrams *et al.* 2002). It is the most common cause of urinary incontinence in the United Kingdom and represents approximately half of all incontinent women (Hannestad *et al.* 2000), with a further 30–40% complaining of mixed symptoms of stress and urge incontinence. An epidemiological survey of 29,500 households across four European countries showed that stress incontinence is the commonest presenting symptom with 42% of respondents admitting to stress-type incontinence in the preceding 30 days (Hunskaar *et al.* 2004). Some 35% of all the women that responded reported any involuntary loss of urine in the preceding 30 days. Approximately half of all women with SUI are slightly bothered and one-third of them are moderately to extremely bothered by their symptoms (Fultz 2003).

Although the symptom of stress incontinence is simplistic in itself, it is frequently accompanied by other urinary symptoms creating an often complex set of symptoms. Proportions of stress, urge and mixed incontinence can be difficult to estimate because of the different assessment of types by authors of epidemiological studies. It has been suggested that mixed incontinence may be over-reported, which may indicate that a larger number of women than has been reported may have pure stress incontinence (Sandvik 1995). Although the use of urodynamic testing has limitations in establishing prevalence of the different types of urinary incontinence, it has repeatedly been shown its value over assessment of symptoms alone in diagnostic accuracy (Jarvis *et al.* 1980). Interestingly, only 39% of women complaining of stress incontinence have urodynamic stress incontinence (Abrams 1983).

Conflicting outcomes of research studies can often be confusing. What remains clear is that it is very important that these women are comprehensively assessed and investigated.

Advanced nursing assessment

Advanced nursing assessment in secondary care links very closely to advanced medical care and in reality there is little that separates the two. The difference between primary and secondary nursing assessment in SUI will primarily be access and proficiency in urodynamic investigation. A specialist nurse should be able to plan, perform and interpret an array of investigations from simple urinalysis to cystometry, ambulatory urodynamic monitoring and possibly video cystourethrography. Nurses have been repeatedly extending their clinical roles and many nurse specialists are now able to perform quite complex investigations on women with SUI that were once performed by the doctor. Additionally, it would not be uncommon to instigate a management plan. Nowadays, the assessment and investigative process should ideally be a multidisciplinary one, including nurses and doctors, as well as other healthcare professionals such as physiotherapists.

Appropriate assessment before any therapy is paramount if treatment is to be tailored to the individual sufferer of SUI and prove successful. This will include a detailed history of her condition, including the onset of her complaint, when it happens, its frequency and severity and how it has affected her life. Appropriate and validated quality-of-life instruments are very useful in assessing the impact of this condition on the patient.

Urinary symptoms

Stress incontinence has been defined as the involuntary loss of urine on effort or exertion, or on sneezing or coughing. It is not associated with urinary urgency and is generally associated with smaller volume loss than urge incontinence. Urinary frequency, however, may develop because of the woman's attempt to minimise urinary leakage by regularly emptying her bladder. Leakage during sexual intercourse tends to be more associated with penetration as opposed to orgasm, which is more associated with overactive bladder (Kelleher *et al.* 1992). Women with stress incontinence may have concomitant voiding dysfunction which may have an impact on treatment outcomes and should therefore be questioned and investigated. Equally, overflow may present as stress incontinence.

It is important to use simple, non-medical language. Many women will deny 'incontinence', but commonly admit to the 'occasional leak'.

Question examples
- Do you ever leak urine?
- Do you leak urine when you cough/sneeze/exercise?
- Do you have to rush to the toilet?
- Do you have to go to the toilet frequently?
- Do you get up at night to pass urine?
- Do you have strain to pass water or feel that you have not emptied your bladder?
- Do you have pain on passing water?

A full account of the patient's medical, drug, surgical, obstetric and gynaecological history should be taken. Though stress incontinence may be demonstrated on clinical examination, it only confirms a symptom and therefore requires further investigation. Anything that causes a high intra-abdominal pressure, such as a large fibroid, obesity or pregnancy, can cause stress incontinence. Additionally, the pressure of constipation or faecal impaction on the pelvic floor can bring about stress incontinence.

Urinary tract infections cause dysuria, frequency, urgency and can lead to incontinence even in fit people who normally have no bladder problems.

Common drugs can affect bladder function, with the most obvious being diuretics. A swift diuresis can have catastrophic results, particularly in the elderly or less mobile. Alpha-adrenoreceptor blocking drugs such as doxazosin and prazosin, can contribute to deterioration in symptoms of stress incontinence (Marshall & Beevers 1996). Other drugs affecting bladder function include tricyclic-antidepressants, sedatives, caffeine and alcohol.

Concomitant diseases, which affect bladder function include endocrine disorders such as diabetes, which can affect peripheral nerves resulting in neuropathy of the bladder; oestrogen deficiency in women; and pituitary disorders. It is not unusual for urinary symptoms to be the first sign of a neurological disorder, such as multiple sclerosis, so it is important to ask about neurological symptoms (e.g. leg weakness and tingling sensations).

Mobility, environment and mental awareness become of paramount importance in an assessment of urinary symptoms.

Biochemical tests

Dipstick urine testing will give a relatively good indication of infection, although a sample of urine should be sent to the laboratory for culture and sensitivity. The presence of a urinary tract infection may invalidate results obtained from urodynamic testing and therefore must be excluded before investigation. Haematuria, dehydration (high specific gravity), urine acidity and diabetes (glucose) can also be easily indicated.

The frequency volume chart

While a clinical interview will provide information regarding voiding and leakage patterns, it is largely subjective and to some extent retrospective. There is a tendency to exaggerate urinary symptoms (Wyman *et al.* 1988) and patients' recollection of incontinent episodes may not be reliable. A self-completed frequency volume chart (FVC) can allow an excellent measure of drinking, voiding and leakage patterns (Figure 6.1). It can provide information concerning frequency, incontinent episodes and the volume of urine voided, which in turn will give an idea of functional bladder capacity. Additionally, it can be sent to patients to complete before their appointment. A complete fluid balance can be assessed over a 24 hour period, if the chart is accurately filled in. An excessively low or high fluid intake will be quickly recognised. FVCs are also a simple objective tool in the assessment of treatment

KING'S College LONDON Founded 1829

King's College Hospital London

Frequency Volume Chart

Time	Day 1 In	Day 1 Out	Day 1 Wet	Day 2 In	Day 2 Out	Day 2 Wet	Day 3 In	Day 3 Out	Day 3 Wet
7 am	200	200	X	200	300	X			
8 am	250			250			200	200	
9 am							250		
10 am								100	
11 am					100				
12 pm	150	150		150			200		
1 pm	150				150		200		
2 pm					100			100	
3 pm					220				
4 pm	250	120		250				50	
5 pm									
6 pm					250	X			
7 pm	150			120			200	300	X
8 pm	150	150	X	100	250		150		
9 pm									
10 pm		200						150	
11 pm					300				
12 am									
1 am									
2 am									
3 am									
4 am									
5 am									
6 am									

Figure 6.1 Frequency Volume Chart

progress or cure. Additional information that can be collected, such as pad usage, associated events and magnitude of leakage will vary, however, from one chart to another. It is really up to the clinician to decide which chart will be most appropriate. When comparing five different charts, Bailey *et al.* (1990) found good acceptability in recording associated events and provocative manoeuvres. Abrams and Klevmark (1996) advocate the use of a 7-day diary to cover both work and leisure periods, but the optimum duration of the FVC is still argued. Clinicians need to exercise care when asking women to complete a diary for a long period of time given that it can be inconvenient and possibly reduce the reliability of the recordings. Common practice is to use a 5-day chart, although some would suggest only three days. The results obtained in each week of a two week diary have been compared (Wyman *et al.* 1988) and there is a strong correlation between the two weeks suggesting that seven days is certainly an acceptable alternative to fourteen. Larsson and Victor (1988) suggested that a short urinary diary of only two days could probably suffice in establishing a pattern of voiding behaviour. In later studies, Larsson *et al.* reported on the reliability of voiding diaries in women with detrusor overactivity (1991) and urodynamic stress incontinence (1992). However, there was great overlap in both diagnostic categories and asymptomatic women. In symptomatic women, it is not possible to reliably distinguish women with urodynamic stress incontinence from those with other urodynamic diagnoses using a FVC alone. Indeed, the FVC has been shown not to be a substitute for cystometry in the investigation of women with urinary incontinence (Tincello & Richmond 1998).

Physical examination

Physical examination should include a vaginal examination to assess for general tissue status and presence of atrophy and/or prolapse, and a bimanual to exclude pelvic masses including uterine pathology, such as fibroids, which can exacerbate SUI. Excoriation or soreness to the perineal area can give some indication to the severity of the problem or whether incorrect continence products are being used. Stress incontinence may be seen if the patient is asked to cough. This is defined by the ICS as the observation of involuntary leakage from the urethra, synchronous with exertion/effort, or sneezing or coughing.

Determining the strength of the pelvic floor musculature will be important in ascertaining starting points for pelvic floor therapy. Consideration needs to be given to specificity, overload and reversibility to achieve an improvement to pelvic floor muscle function (DiNubile 1991). *Specificity* considers using the correct muscles in a functional way, *overload* is concerned with working muscles harder that what would normally be required and *reversibility* is reverting muscles back to a lesser ability unless they are sustained with correct exercise.

Any uncertainty about a patient's neurological status requires further investigation of muscle, sensory and motor function.

Pad testing

Pad testing will verify and quantify the degree of urine loss; however, it does not give a diagnosis. It was first described by Sutherst *et al.* (1981) and subsequently modified and accepted by the standardisation committee of the International Continence Society (ICS) in 1988 (Abrams *et al.* 1988). The recommendation is that the subject has a fluid load of 500 ml before the test, which lasts for 1 hour. There are some variations, however, in test time and some investigators instil a standard volume (usually 250 ml) into the bladder.

The pad (or device) is weighed before the test and then again after the set time which usually contains some standard provocative manoeuvres (e.g. coughing and hand washing). Anything below 1 g is considered insignificant, as this may be caused by perspiration or vaginal discharge (Sutherst *et al*. 1981). More recently, this has been found to be less than 0.3 g in 24 hours (Karantanis *et al*. 2003). Home pad testing is considered less controlled, lasting from 24 to 48 hours, but generally has a better reproducibility (Lose & Versi 1992).

More recent studies have looked at the repeatability of pad testing. Karantanis *et al*. (2005) assessed the repeatability of the home pad test and found that a single 24-hour pad test correlated highly with a 7 day average and was considered sufficient to gauge severity of leakage. The one-hour pad test shows poor repeatability and although is a useful baseline measure of incontinence it is not considered an optimal measure of post-treatment change (Simons *et al*. 2001). When the two pad tests are compared, little relationship to underlying urodynamic diagnoses on either type was found. The 24-hour pad appears to be more clinically useful than the one-hour pad test (Matharu *et al*. 2004) and therefore questions the clinical use of the one-hour pad test altogether. It has been suggested that asking women whether she is continent of urine may be as good as performing a one-hour pad test. (Abdel-fattah *et al*. 2004)

Uroflowmetry

Uroflowmetry is simple, non-invasive and provides an objective measurement of voiding ability. It is particularly pertinent to women complaining of voiding dysfunction and was first described by von Garretts in 1956. It measures the volume of urine voided, maximum flow rate, acceleration to maximum flow, time to maximum flow, flow time and average flow time (Figure 6.2). A normal flow rate is bell-shaped in appearance (Figure 6.3) and with a voided volume of greater than 150 ml should have a maximum flow rate of greater than 15 ml/s. Urinary flow rate and voided volume does, however, vary significantly with age and sex (von Garretts 1956). Nomograms have been established to provide a normal reference range of volumes voided for both women and men (Haylen *et al*. 1989). The cause of voiding difficulties cannot be identified by uroflowmetry alone and simultaneous recording

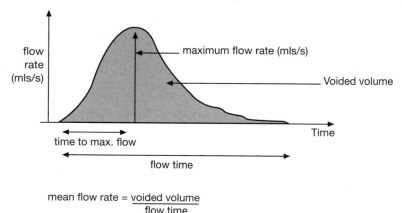

Figure 6.2 Uroflowmetry information

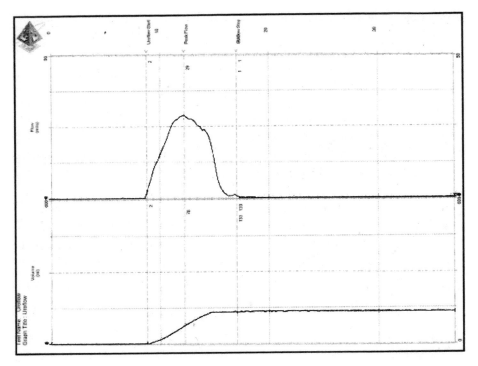

Figure 6.3 Normal Flow-rate

of detrusor pressure will need to be recorded to differentiate a hypotonic detrusor or outflow obstruction. Equally, a normal flow rate does not exclude voiding pathology (Pauwels *et al.* 2005), and a normal non-intubated uroflow (free-flow) does not necessarily exclude an abnormal pressure flow study (Defreitas *et al.* 2003).

Women with stress incontinence however appear to void at a lower detrusor pressure (Lemack *et al.* 2002).

It is usual to measure a post micturition residual of urine following voiding, either by ultrasound or catheterisation (less than 50 ml is normal). This is particularly important in women with symptoms suggestive of voiding difficulties, those who require continence surgery or pharmacological therapy that may exacerbate voiding difficulties.

Cystometry

The measurement of pressure–volume relation within the bladder was first described in 1882, by Mosso and Pellacani. This type of measurement, commonly known as simple cystometry, however, is not altogether accurate as it presumes intravesical pressure is detrusor pressure. It was not until the early 1970s that this test became clinically useful with the introduction of pressure transducers and accurate chart recorders, which were able to electronically subtract abdominal pressure from intravesical pressure, thus giving a true detrusor pressure. The International Continence Society (ICS) has produced guidelines on good practice for urodynamics (Shafer *et al.* 2002).

Subtracted cystometry (Figure 6.4) measures the pressures within the bladder during filling and voiding. It involves passing a filling catheter (this can also be used to measure post-micturition residual following initial uroflowmetry), a pressure transducer into the bladder, and a pressure transducer into the rectum (or vagina) to measure intra-abdominal activity. Intravesical and abdominal pressure can then be recorded simultaneously resulting in the subtracted detrusor pressure.

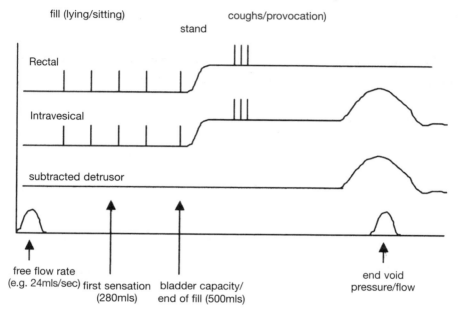

Figure 6.4 Diagrammatic representation of a normal cystometric trace

Physiological bladder filling is around 100 ml/h. During retrograde cystometry, the bladder is filled (filling phase) with saline, with the patient either supine or sitting. A filling rate of 100 ml/min is common (fast-fill). First bladder sensation and bladder capacity is recorded. A normal first bladder sensation is between 150 and 250 ml and a normal bladder capacity is between 400 and 600 ml. During filling (to 500 ml), the detrusor pressure should not normally rise above 15 cm H_2O. A rise greater than this will indicate a non-compliant bladder. Low compliance (Figure 6.5) is only demonstrated during fast filling of the bladder and can be associated with chronic inflammation, post radiotherapy fibrosis or following long term catheterisation, although many cases are idiopathic (Coolsaet 1985).

Any uninhibited spontaneous detrusor contractions during the filling phase indicate systolic detrusor overactivity, and if they occur on provocation, they indicate

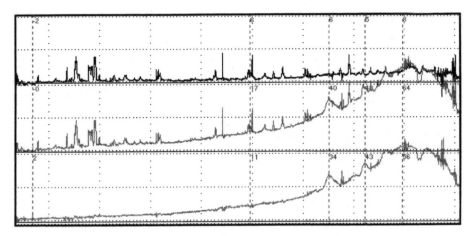

Figure 6.5 Low compliance and systolic detrusor overactivity

provoked detrusor overactivity. These are particularly useful to note, as they will often create a symptom of stress incontinence.

Once the bladder is filled, the subject then stands up (or sits) and the filling catheter is removed. While standing they are asked to perform a set of provocative manoeuvres, which may include coughing, hand washing or heel bouncing. Any detrusor rise or leakage is noted. Once the required information is obtained, they are asked to pass urine into the flow meter (voiding phase). Simultaneous detrusor pressure readings can then be recorded in relation to the urinary flow (pressure-flow study).

Urodynamic stress incontinence is noted during filling cystometry and is defined as the involuntary leakage of urine during increased abdominal pressure in the absence of a detrusor contraction (Abrams *et al.* 2002). On a cystometric trace it is not possible to identify incontinence unless the trace is annotated (Figure 6.6).

Studies have repeatedly shown the greater value of urodynamics over assessment of symptoms alone in diagnostic accuracy (Jarvis *et al.* 1980; James *et al.* 1999), and just 39% of women complaining of stress incontinence have USI demonstrated on cystometry (Abrams 1983).

Although many women may be treated conservatively without invasive investigation, the predictive value of stress symptoms alone is not high enough to serve as a basis for surgical management (Weidner *et al.* 2001; Dwyer 2004). Invasive urodynamic investigations must be tailored to the individual patient, as there should ideally be no barriers on who has access to investigation for stress incontinence.

Summary

Stress incontinence is a debilitating condition which adversely affects the lives of women. Although an assessment of symptoms, examination and a frequency volume

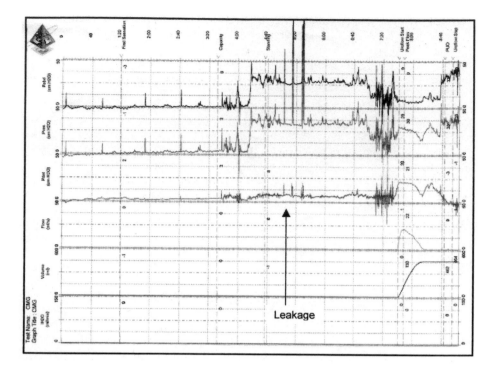

Leakage

Figure 6.6 Urodynamic stress incontinence

chart may all indicate stress incontinence, a diagnosis of urodynamic stress incontinence can only be made after cystometric tests are performed to exclude detrusor overactivity.

By the time women are seen within the secondary care setting, and particularly a tertiary referral centre, they may well have seen a host of other healthcare professionals. Others may have only seen their general practitoner and obtained a simple referral. The specialist nurse must spend the time she/he has efficiently to establish relevant details to allow an appropriate assessment in order to tailor effective treatment. They are in a unique role to use their knowledge and skills to help women with stress incontinence. They should, however, not work in isolation but with a multidisciplinary approach to maximise patient benefit. This should involve primary care services, thus creating integrated continence services (Department of Health 2000).

References

Abdel-fattah, M., Barrington J.W. & Youssef, M. (2004). The standard 1-hour pad test: does it have any value in clinical practice? *European Urology* **46**, 377–380.

Abrams, P. The clinical contribution of urodynamics. (1983). In *Urodynamics* (ed.) Abrams P., Feneley, R. & Torrens M., pp. 118–174. Berlin: Springer-Verlag.

Abrams, P., Blaivas, J. G., Stanton, S. L. & Andersen, J. T. (1988). The standardisation of terminology of lower urinary tract function. *Scandinavian Journal of Urology and Nephrology. Supplementum* **114**, 5–19.

Abrams, P., & Klemark, B. (1996). Frequency volume charts: an indispensable part of lower urinary tract assessment. *Scandinavian Journal of Urology and Nephrology. Supplementum* **179**, 47–53.

Abrams, P., Cardozo, L., Fall, M., Griffiths, D., Rosier, P., Ulmsten, J., van Keirebroek, P., Victor, A. & Wein, A. (2002). The standardisation of Terminology of Lower Urinary Tract Function: Report from the Standardisation Sub-Committee of the International Continence Society. *Neurourology and Urodynamics* **21**, 167–178.

Bailey, R., Sephaerd, A. & Tribe, B. (1990). How information can be obtained from frequency/volume charts? *Neurourology and Urodynamics* **9**, 382–383.

Coolsaet, B. (1985). Bladder compliance and detrusor activity during the collection phase. *Neurourology and Urodynamics* **4**, 263–273.

Defreitas, G. A., Lemack, G. E. & Zimmerman, P.E. (2003). Nonintubated uroflowmetry as a predictor of normal pressure flow study in women with stress incontinence. *Urology* **62**, 905–908.

Department of Health (2000). *Good Practice in Continence Services*. London: Department of Health.

DiNubile, N. A. (1991). Strength training. *Clinics in Sports Medicine* **10**, 33–62.

Dwyer, P. L. (2004). Differentiating stress urinary incontinence from urge urinary incontinence. *International Journal of Gynaecology and Obstetrics*. **86** (Suppl. 1), S17–S24.

Fultz, N.H., Burgio, Diokno, A. C., Kinchen, K. S., Obenchain, R. & Bump, R.C. (2003). Burden of stress urinary incontinence for community-dwelling women. *American Journal of Obstetrics and Gynecology* **189**, 1275–1282.

Haylen, B. T., Ashby, D., Sutherst, J. R, Frazer, M. I. & West, C. R. (1989). Maximum and average flow rates in normal male and female populations – the Liverpool nomograms. *British Journal of Urology* **64**, 30–38.

Hannestad, Y. S., Rortveit, G., Sandvik, H. & Hunskaar, S. (2000). A community-based epidemiological survey of female urinary incontinence: the Norwegian EPINCONT study. Epidemiology of incontinence in the County of Nord-Trondelag. *Journal of Clinical Epidemiology* **53**, 1150–1157.

Hunskaar, S., Lose, G., Sykes, D. & Voss, S. (2004). The prevalence of urinary incontinence in women in four European countries. *BJU International* **93**, 324–330.

James, M., Jackson, S., Shepherd, A. & Abrams, P. (1999). Pure stress leakage symptomatology: is it safe to discount detrusor instability? *British Journal of Obstetrics and Gynaecology* **106**, 1255–1258.

Jarvis, G. J., Hall, S., Stamp, S. & Millar, D. R. (1980). An assessment of urodynamic investigation in incontinent women. *British Journal of Obstetrics and Gynaecology* **87**, 873–896.

Karantanis, E., O'Sullivan, R. & Moore, K. H. (2003). The 24-hour pad test in continent women and men: normal values and cyclical alterations. *British Journal of Obstetrics and Gynaecology* **110**, 567–571.

Karantanis, E., Allen, W., Stevermuer, T. L., Simons, A. M., O'Sullivan, R. & Moore, K. H. (2005). The repeatability of the 24-hour pad test. *International Urogynecology Journal and Pelvic Floor Dysfunction* **16**, 63–68.

Kelleher, C. J., Cardozo, L.D., Wise, B. G. & Cutner, A. (1992). The impact of urinary incontinence on sexual function. *Neurourology and Urodynamics* **11**, 359–360.

Larsson, G. & Victor, A. (1988). Micturition patterns in a healthy female population, studied with a frequency volume chart. *Scandinavian Journal of Urology and Nephrology. Supplementum* **114**, 53–57.

Larsson, G., Abrams, P. & Victor, A. (1991). The frequency/volume chart in detrusor instability. *Neurourology and Urodynamics* **10**, 533–543.

Larsson, G. & Victor, A. (1992). The frequency/volume chart in genuine stress incontinent women. *Neurourology and Urodynamics* **11**, 23–31.

Lemack, G. E., Baseman, A. G. & Zimmern, P. E. (2002). Voiding dynamics: a comparison of pressure-flow studies between asymptomatic and incontinent women. *Urology* **59**, 42–46.

Lose, G. & Versi, E. (1992). Pad weighing tests in the diagnosis and quantification of incontinence. *International Urogynaecology Journal* **3**, 324–328.

Marshall, H. L. & Beevers, D. G. (1996). Alpha-adrenoreceptor blocking drugs and female urinary incontinence: prevalence and reversibility. *British Journal of Clinical Pharmacology* **42**, 507–509.

Matharu, G. S., Assassa, R. P., Williams, K. S., Donaldson, M., Matthes, R., Tincello, D. G. & Mayne, C. J. (2004). Objective assessment of urinary incontinence in women: comparison of the one-hour and 24-hour pad tests. *European Urology* **45**, 208–212.

Mosso, A. & Pellacani, P. (1882). sur les functions de la vessie. Methode de recherché. *Archives italiennes de biologie* **1**, 97–128.

Pauwels, E., de Wacchter, S. & Wyndaele, J. J. (2005). A normal flow pattern in women does not exclude voiding pathology. *International Urogynecology Journal and Pelvic Floor Dysfunction* **16**, 104–108.

Sandvik, H., Hunskaar, S., Vanvik, A., Bratt, H., Seim, A. & Hernstad, R. (1995). Diagnostic classification of female urinary incontinence: an epidemiological survey corrected for validity. *Journal of Clinical Epidemiology* **48**, 339–343.

Schafer, W., Abrams, P., Liao, L., Mattiasson, A., Pesce, F., Spangberg, A., Sterling, A. M., Zinner, N. R. & van Kerrebroeck, P. (2002). Report on Good Urodynamic Practice. *Neurourology and Urodynamics* **21**, 261–274.

Simons AM, Yoong WC, Buckland S, Moore KH. (2001). Inadequate repeatability of the one-hour pad test: the need for a new incontinence outcome measure. *British Journal of Obstetrics and Gynaecology* **108**, 315–319.

Sutherst, J., Brown, M. & Shawler, M. (1981). Assessing the severity of urinary incontinence in women by weighing perineal pads. *Lancet* **1**, 1128–1130.

Tincello DG, Richmon DH (1998). The Larsson frequency/volume chart is not a substitute for cystometry in investigation of women with urinary incontinence. *International Urogynecology Journal and Pelvic Floor Dysfunction* **9**, 391–396.

von Garretts, B. (1956). Analysis of micturition: a new method of recording the voiding of the bladder. *Acta Chirurgica Scandinavica* **112**, 326–340.

Weidner, A. C., Myers, E. R., Visco, A. G., Cundiff, G. W. & Bump, R. C. (2001). Which women with stress incontinence require urodynamic evaluation? *American Journal of Obsterics and Gynecology* **184**, 20–27.

Wyman JF, Sung CC, Harkins SW, Wilson MS, Fantl JA. (1988). The urinary diary in the evaluation of incontinent women: a test retest analysis. *Obstetrics and Gynecology* **71**, 812–817.

Chapter 7

Secondary medical investigations for urinary incontinence

Charlotte Chaliha and Vik Khullar

Introduction

General recommendations for evaluating women with uncomplicated urinary incontinence include a detailed history, physical examination, urinalysis and, if possible, assessment of postvoid residual. Further investigations for secondary care are usually reserved for those with complicating factors or co-morbidities. However, this basic evaluation performed in the primary care setting, and the basis for which empirical therapy is instituted, may lead to inappropriate treatment due to inaccurate diagnosis, especially as history often has a poor relationship to underlying pathology (Jarvis *et al.* 1980; Handa *et al.* 1995).

There are a variety of investigations for lower urinary tract dysfunction, as shown in Table 7.1. Not all patients require such detailed investigation and assessment techniques should be tailored to the individual patient. Appropriate use of these tests provides useful information on which to base treatment and this is essential if instituting surgical treatment.

Table 7.1 Investigations for lower urinary tract dysfunction

Non-specialist investigations	History
	Examination
	Midstream urine
	Frequency–volume chart
	Postvoid residual
Specialist investigations	Uroflowmetry
	Cystometry
	Video-cystometry
	Ambulatory urodynamics
	Urethral pressure profilometry
	Intravenous urography
	Micturating cystography
	Ultrasonography
	Magnetic resonance imaging

Specialist investigations

Pad tests

Pad tests are used to quantify the degree of urine lost so allowing objective evaluation of severity of leakage and effect of treatment in a non-invasive way. There are also specially designed pads that allow detection of urine during ambulatory monitoring.

The pad tests can be divided into those less than 1 h, 1 h, 24 h and 48 h. The short pad tests (less than 1 h and 1 h) have not been found to be good in assessing the severity of urinary incontinence (Mundt-Pettersen *et al.* 1984; Lose *et al.* 1986). The reproducibility of the 1 h pad test is improved by using a standardised bladder volume and a provocative exercise regime. The 24- and 48 h pad tests have better sensitivity and reproducibility (Jorgensen *et al.* 1987; Versi *et al.* 1996) and the difference between the two is minimal such that a pad test of over 24 h is not required. A pad test weight gain of ≥ 4 g/24 h is a positive test. The amount of urine lost during the test is determined by the change of weight of the pad. A weight gain of greater than 1 g signifies incontinence. Although the pad test cannot distinguish between detrusor overactivity and urodynamic stress incontinence, it can indicate severity of incontinence and is a relatively simple and inexpensive test. Apart from the purchase of pads, the only other costs are a weighing machine. If pads are going to be used, the pad test protocol should be standardised with clear instructions to the patient.

Urodynamics

The basic urodynamic equipment consists of uroflowmetry and cystometry. It can be purchased individually or as a complete system. Most modern machines consist of a computerised system with a computer screen to visualise the investigation as it occurs. Event markers can record events as they occur, with simultaneous recording of measurements. The trace can be stored and so reviewed at a later date if required. A paper print out can also be generated for storage in notes. These systems are useful particularly in research settings.

Uroflowmetry

Uroflowmetry is an essential part of the urodynamic investigation as a screening test for voiding difficulties. It enables the measurement of maximum flow rate, average flow rate, flow time and time to maximum flow. Its major advantage is that it can identify women with poor peak flow. However, it cannot distinguish between outflow obstruction and detrusor hypotonia.

The patient should be asked to attend with a full bladder and the flowmeter placed where voiding can occur in privacy. There are several commercial flowmeters of which those that use the principles of weight transduction, a rotating disc and capacitance transducer are the best known and most well validated. The weight transducer flowmeter weighs the volume voided, over the time voided, to record a change in the volume voided over time. It therefore measures a change in mass and so needs to be calibrated with fluid of the correct density. The rotating disc meter depends on a servometer maintaining the rotation of the disc at a constant speed. As urine hits the disc, extra power is required to maintain the speed and this is converted into an electronic signal. They have the advantage that they do not require priming with fluid. The capacitance flowmeter is the simplest and consists of a funnel that leads into a collecting vessel. A transducer is attached that dips into the vessel.

All three types are accurate enough for clinical use although an independent assessment of flowmeters found that the rotating disc device is the most accurate (Rowan *et al.* 1987).

Cystometry

Ideally, all patients with lower urinary tract symptoms should undergo cystometry for accurate diagnosis and treatment as the bladder is an unreliable witness (Jarvis *et al.* 1980; Larg-Jansseen *et al.* 1991). We suggest urodynamics should be performed in those patients:

- Planned for continence surgery
- Those with a recurrent symptoms after previous continence surgery
- Those with mixed symptoms
- Those with voiding dysfunction
- After failure of empirical therapy

During cystometry, the pressure–volume relation of the bladder is measured and also detrusor contractility, bladder sensation and compliance.

Cystometry should be performed in the upright position as this is more physiological and is when the majority of patients complain of symptoms. The filling medium should be water or 0.9% saline at room or body temperature. Ice-cold fluid can stimulate bladder contractility and should not be used (Aslund *et al.* 1988). Three filling rates have been described by the International Continence Society (ICS) (Abrams *et al.* 1988):

- Slow fill at 10 ml/min
- Medium fill at 10–100 ml/min
- Fast fill when the rate is greater than 100 ml/min

Fast filling is provocative for patients with detrusor overactivity although will not 'provoke' a stable bladder to contract (Arnold *et al.* 1974; Ramsden *et al.* 1977). During the test the patient should stand and provocations such as heel bouncing and coughing should occur (Bates *et al.* 1970). Any rises in detrusor pressure may be observed and noted if associated with urgency. At the end of filling, the filling catheter is removed and the patient is asked to void into a flowmeter. The maximum voiding pressure and flow rate can then be noted. This can distinguish a patient with detrusor hypotonia (low pressure and low flow) from one with obstructed flow (high pressure and low flow). Any postvoid residual can be measured at the end of flow. Evaluation of pressure flow parameters has high reproducibility and consistency in evaluating lower urinary tract function during voiding (Digesu *et al.* 2003) and can provide prognostic information regarding the likelihood of developing voiding dysfunction postoperatively (Gateau *et al.* 2003; Miller *et al.* 2003; Wang & Chen 2003).

Multi-channel cystometry requires a urine flowmeter, an electronic device to subtract abdominal from vesical pressure, a recorder with print out and an amplifying unit. The bladder pressure can be measured with either a fluid catheter connected to an external pressure transducer or a solid microtip transducer mounted onto a solid 7F catheter. Abdominal pressure can be measured with a rectal catheter, or vaginal catheter if this is not possible.

There are, therefore, variations in technique, and each unit should aim to standardise its procedure so comparisons can be made over time.

Videocystometry

This can be considered to be the gold standard for lower urinary tract investigation (Benness *et al.* 1989). The use of radio-opaque medium allows visualisation during cystometry with X-ray screening and is said to be more sensitive in the diagnosis of urodynamic stress incontinence than simple cystometry. The lower urinary tract is visualised while there is synchronous recording of bladder function. The diagnostic criteria for intrinsic sphincter deficiency is the presence of funnelling (an open bladder neck and proximal urethra) with subsequent leakage of urine/contrast with rises in abdominal pressure without a detrusor-pressure rise. However, it should be noted that observation of contrast medium leaking into the proximal urethra without associated bladder contraction has been seen in 50% of continent women (Versi *et al.* 1986).

The unit will require X-ray facilities to allow for imaging and trained radiology staff. If urodynamic equipment is not available with X-ray imaging it may need to be moved and this increases the risk of breakages and damage to the systems. All staff operating X-ray equipment need to have training and certification in safe usage. It is more time consuming than simple cystometry and more expensive. It is not necessary in every patient as simpler studies can often provide the diagnosis. However, in cases where the history does not fit the diagnosis, where there has been previous surgical intervention or a history of neurological abnormality, it can be useful and the cost justified (Bates & Corney 1971; McGuire & Brady 1979). Videocystourethrography can also visualise bladder or urethral diverticulae, urethral stenosis or vesicoureteric reflux which may be present in up to 7% of incontinent patients (Benness *et al.* 1989; Shepherd 1990).

Ambulatory urodynamic monitoring

This is most commonly used as a second-line test and aims to investigate the bladder under more physiological conditions and when laboratory urodynamics do not match symptoms. The ambulatory systems have three main components: the transducers, recording system and analysing system. Solid-state intravesical and rectal transducers are used. The recording system should be portable and battery operated. The recording system should also have the facility to be connected to an electronic nappy and flowmeter.

Additional to the costs of the ambulatory equipment, a computer is required to review and download the traces. A normal protocol for ambulatory urodynamics lasts 4 h and during this time the patient is asked to drink normally and keep a detailed diary of symptoms and events. Provocative manoeuvres are carried out with the bladder full every half hour. The catheter position needs to be checked after each void or leak. It is, therefore, time consuming and useful only in a unit with appropriate manpower and training to provide this service.

There is conflicting evidence regarding the usefulness of ambulatory testing. Although it may be thought to be more sensitive and physiological than laboratory urodynamics (Van Waalwijk van Dorn *et al.* 1991; Hill *et al.* 1995), it may overdiagnose detrusor overactivity. Studies of asymptomatic subjects show 38–69% have detrusor overactivity on ambulatory testing, but only 18% on laboratory urodynamics (Van Waalwijk van Dorn *et al.* 1992; Robertson *et al.* 1994; Heslington & Hilton 1995). It is very useful for voiding problems where a pressure–flow study cannot be obtained during a laboratory urodynamic test as the woman would void at least four times during the four hours. Detecting stress incontinence is reduced with ambulatory urodynamics due to the reduced bladder volume during provocation.

Urethral pressure profilometry

The pressure profile is usually performed using microtip transducers and balloon catheters. The microtip transducers are relatively expensive and fragile and are attached to a pull through system that must be compatible with the existing urodynamic machine. A soft silicone catheter with two transducers 6 cm apart is gradually withdrawn along the urethra allowing simultaneous recording of urethral and vesical pressure. From subtraction of these measurements, urethral pressure can be derived.

Urethral pressure profilometry is not required in all patients, but should be considered in those with voiding difficulties and those with previous failed surgery as a low maximum urethral closure pressure (< 20 cm H_2O) has been considered predictive of poor outcome of conventional surgery and is a strong indicator of intrinsic sphincter deficiency (Sand *et al.* 1987).

The maximum urethral pressure and maximum urethral closure pressure are reduced in women with urodynamic stress incontinence compared to controls (Hilton & Stanton 1983; Versi 1990); however, there is a wide overlap in values making this of limited value in distinguishing these groups of patients. A high maximum urethral closure pressure indicates obstruction and in these cases a urethrotomy may be considered. It may also be of use in diagnosing urethral diverticula (Bhatia *et al.* 1981).

Radiology of the lower urinary tract

Imaging of the lower urinary tract is increasingly used as an adjunct to urodynamic studies and has the advantage that it allows evaluation of the lower urinary tract and its surrounding structures.

X-ray

Anteroposterior and lateral images of the spinal cord are used to identify vertebral defects in patients suspected of having neurogenic incontinence, especially if there are associated abnormalities on neurogenic examination. Increased visualisation of the lower urinary tract is possible with the use of contrast agents, such as videocystourethrography as described. Contrast instilled at the time of urodynamics may allow visualisation of diverticula, fistula, stones, tumours and reflux.

Ultrasound

Ultrasound can be used to visualise fluid-filled structures without the use of contrast medium and so has the advantage of avoiding ionising radiation. It allows the visualisation of soft tissues such as the kidney, urethra, urethral sphincter and bladder wall. The bony enclosure of the pelvis limits ultrasound imaging to the transabdominal, transvaginal, transrectal and transperineal approaches. Each approach has its advantages and limitations. The type of probe and frequency of the ultrasound wave (1–10 mHz) emitted determines which tissues are seen and the quality of the image obtained. The higher the ultrasound frequency, the better the resolution of the image, although an increased frequency has reduced depth of penetration due to increased attenuation.

Vaginal and abdominal ultrasound is routinely used for measuring residual bladder volumes. A portable bladder volume scanner is useful for nursing staff assessment of residual volume, both for outpatient management but also for inpatient care and reduces the risk of urinary tract infection from catheterisation. Ultrasound can image diverticula and associated transitional cell carcinoma and calculi are seen in 5% of cases (Fox *et al.* 1962). Transabdominal imaging does not allow visualisation of the bladder neck as this is obstructed by the pubic symphysis. Transvaginal ultrasound allows imaging of the bladder and periurethral structures as the probe is closer to relevant structures. The urethral sphincter can be seen as an ovoid structure around the urethra. However, as the probe distorts the urethra it is not good for assessing bladder neck movement of urinary leakage during rises in intra-abdominal pressure (Wise *et al.* 1992). Translabial and transrectal imaging have been suggested as alternatives as they do not distort vaginal and urethral anatomy. In neurological patients with decreased or absent anal sensation, transrectal imaging may be of particular use, although with complete spinal cord transection insertion of the probe into the anal canal may alter sacral cord reflexes. The bladder neck and proximal urethra can be visualised with transrectal ultrasound during voiding for which there are specially designed chairs and these images are similar to those obtained with videocystourethrography (Shapero *et al.* 1983).

Bladder wall thickness can be estimated in a reproducible manner using a perineal or transvaginal probe. This method has good sensitivity as a screening test for detrusor overactivity as long as the bladder empties to less than 20 ml after voiding and if the bladder wall thickness is greater than 5 mm. It has also been shown to be a good second-line test after laboratory urodynamics instead of ambulatory urodynamics in 60% of women.

Three-dimensional ultrasound can be used to assess a specific volume allowing images to be obtained in unlimited number through the selected volume. The urethral sphincter can be defined by this approach and these images correlated well with cadaveric studies (Schaer *et al.* 1998).

Ultrasound imaging is not only limited to the lower urinary tract, but good-quality images of the pelvic floor can be obtained. The levator ani hiatus and surface area are altered in women after vaginal delivery and in those with prolapse (Athansiou *et al.* 1996; Toozs-Hobson *et al.* 1997; Delancey & Hurd 1998).

Magnetic resonance imaging

Static, dynamic and three-dimensional imaging Magnetic Resonance Imaging (MRI) studies have enhanced the understanding of pelvic floor anatomy (Fielding *et al.* 2000; Goh *et al.* 2000). The advantages of MRI include no requirement for urethral catheterisation and detailed views of the pelvis at rest and during straining. However, it is expensive and at present limited to research use.

Electromyography and nerve conduction studies

These specialised tests may be performed in the investigation of the neurological patient and are often part of the routine diagnostic investigation as well as research tools. They do not have a role in routine clinical practice.

Electrical impulses in muscle fibres are measured during spontaneous activity of neural stimulation. There are two main techniques: surface electromyography (EMG) measures the nerve potential over the skin overlying the specific muscle when the pudendal nerve is stimulated, and single-fibre EMG records nerve activity from individual muscle fibres. More myogenic damage and denervation is seen in patients with intrinsic sphincter deficiency compared to those with stress incontinence and urethral hypermobility (Takahashi *et al.* 2000).

Conclusions

Specialist investigations in secondary care allow thorough evaluation of the incontinent patient to refine diagnosis and treatment. These investigations should be tailored appropriately to the individual patient, and their limitations as well as potential values understood.

*References*_____

Abrams, P., Blaivas, J. G., Stanton, S. L. *et al.* (1988). The International Continence Society Committee on Standardisation of Terminology: the standardisation of terminology of lower urinary tract function. *Scandinavian Journal of Urology and Nephrology. Supplementum* **114**, 5–19.

Arnold, E. P., Brown, A. & Webster, J. (1974). Videocystourethography with synchronous detrusor pressure and flow recording. *Annals of the Royal College of Surgeons* **55**, 99–98.

Aslund, K., Rentzhogh, L. & Sandstromb, G. (1988). Effects of ice-cold saline and acid solution in urodynamics. *Proceedings of the 18th annual meeting of the International Continence Society*, Oslo, Norway, ICS, pp 1–2.

Athansiou, S., Boos, K., Khullar, V., Anders, K. & Cardozo, L. (1996). Pathogenesis of genuine stress incontinence and urogenital prolapse. *Neurourology and Urodynamics* **15**, 339–340.

Bates, C. P. & Corney, L. E. (1971). Synchronous cine/pressure/flow/cystourethography: a method of routine urodynamic investigation. *British Journal of Radiology* **44**, 44–50.

Bates, C. P., Whiteside, C. G. & Turner-Warwick, R. T. (1970). Synchronous cine/pressure/flow/cystourethography with special reference to stress and urge incontinence. *British Journal of Urology* **44**, 44–50.

Benness, C. J., Barnick, C. G. & Cardozo, L. D. (1989). Is there a place for routine videocystourethography in the assessment of lower urinary tract dysfunction? *Neurourology and Urodynamics* **8**, 299–300.

Bergman, A., Ballard, C. A. & Platt, L. D. (1988). Ultrasonic evaluation of urethrovesical junction in women with stress urinary incontinence. *Journal of Clinical Ultrasound* **16**, 295–300.

Bhatia, M. N., McCarthy, T. A. & Ostergard, D. (1981). Urethral diverticula, urethral closure profile: a preliminary report. *Progress in Clinical and Biological Research* **78**, 239–242.

Delancey, J. O. & Hurd, W. W. (1998). Size of the urogenital prolapse in the levator ani muscles in normal women and women with pelvic organ prolapse. *Obstetrics and Gynecology* **91**, 364–368.

Digesu, G. A., Hutchings, A., Salvatore, S., Selvaggi, L. & Khullar, V. (2003). Reproducibility and reliability of pressure flow parameters in women. *British Journal of Obstetrics and Gynaecology* **110**, 774–776.

Fielding, J. R., Dumanli, H., Schreyer, A. G., Okuda, S., Gering, D. T., Zou, K. H., Kikinis, R. & Jolesz, F. A. (2000). MR-based three dimensional modelling of the normal pelvic floor in women: quantification of muscle mass. *American Journal of Roentgenology* **174**, 657–660.

Fox, M., Power, R. F. & Bruce, A. W. (1962). Diverticulum of the bladder: presentation and evaluation in 115 cases. *British Journal of Urology* **34**, 286–289.

Gateau, T., Faramarzi-Roques, R., Le Normand, L. *et al.* (2003). Clinical and urodynamic repercussions after TVT procedure and how to diminish patient complaints. *European Journal of Urology* **44**, 372–376.

Goh, V., Halligan, S., Kaplan, G. *et al.* (2000). Dynamic MR imaging of the pelvic floor in asymptomatic subjects. *American Journal of Roentgenology* **174**, 6661–6666.

Handa, V. L., Jensen, J. K. & Ostergard, D. R. (1995). Federal guidelines for the management of urinary incontinence in the United States. Which patients should undergo urodynamic testing? *International Urogynecology Journal* **6**, 198–203.

Heslington, K. & Hilton, P. (1995). Ambulatory monitoring and conventional cystometry in asymptomatic volunteers. *British Journal of Obstetrics and Gynaecology* **103**, 434–441.

Hill, S., Khullar, V., Cardozo, L., Anders, K. & Yip, A. (1995). Ambulatory urodynamics versus videocystometrogram: a test-retest analysis. *Neurourology and Urodynamics* **14**, 528–529.

Hilton, P. & Stanton, S. L. (1983). Urethral pressure measurement by microtransducer: the results in symptom-free women and in those with genuine stress incontinence. *British Journal of Obstetrics and Gynaecology* **90**, 919–933.

Jarvis, G. J., Hall, S., Stamp, S., Millar, D. R. & Johnson, A. (1980). Assessment of urodynamic examination in continent women. *British Journal of Obstetrics and Gynaecology* **87**, 893–896.

Jorgensen, L., Lose, G. & Thunedborg, B. (1987). One hour pad weighing test for objective assessment of female urinary incontinence. *Obstetrics and Gynecology* **69**, 39–41.

Larg-Jansseen, F. M., Debruyne, F. M. J. & Van Weel, C. (1991). Value of the patients case history in diagnosing urinary incontinence in general practice. *British Journal of Urology* **67**, 569–572.

Lose, G., Gammelgaard, J. & Jorgensen, T. J. (1986). The one-hour pad test: reproducibility and the correlation between the test result, the start volume in the bladder and the diuresis. *Neurourology and Urodynamics* **5**, 17–21.

McGuire, E. J. & Brady, S. (1979). Detrusor sphincter dyssynergia. *Journal of Urology* **121**, 774–777.

Miller, E. A., Amundsen, C. L., Toh, K. L., *et al.* (2003). Pre-operative urodynamic evaluation may predict voiding dysfunction in women undergoing the pubovaginal sling. *Journal of Urology* **169**, 2234–2237.

Mundt-Pettersen, B., Mattiason, A. & Sundin, T. (1984). Reproducibility of the 1 hour incontinence test proposed by the ICS standardisation committee. *Proceedings of the International Continence Society, 14th annual meeting*, Innsbruck: International Continence Society, pp 90–91.

Myers, R. P., Cahill, D. R., Kay, P. A. *et al.* (2000). Puboperineal: muscular boundaries of the male urogenital hiatus in 3D form magnetic resonance imaging. *Journal of Urology* **164**, 1412–1415.

Ramsden, P. D., Smith, J. C., Pierce, J. M. & Ardran, G. M. (1977). The unstable bladder: fact or artefact? *British Journal of Urology* **49**, 633–639.

Robertson, A. S., Griffiths, C. J., Ramsden, P. D. & Neal, D. E. (1994). Bladder function in healthy volunteers: ambulatory monitoring and conventional urodynamic studies. *British Journal of Urology* **73**, 242–249.

Rowan, D., James, E. D., Kramer, A. E. J. L. *et al.* (1987). Urodynamic equipment: technical aspects. International Continence Working Party on Urodynamic Equipment. *Journal of Medical Engineering and Technology* **11**, 57–64.

Sand, P. K., Bowen, L. W., Panganiban, R. & Ostergard, D. R. (1987). The low pressure urethra as a factor in failed retropubic surgery. *Obstetrics and Gynecology* **68**, 399–402.

Schaer, G. N., Schmid, T., Peschers, U. & Delancey, J. O. (1998). Intraurethral ultrasound correlated with urethral histology. *Obstetrics and Gynecology* **91**, 60–64.

Shapero, L. G., Friedland, G. W. & Perkash, I. (1983). Transrectal sonographic voiding cystourethography: studies in neuromuscular bladder dysfunction. *American Journal of Roentgenology* **141**, 83–90.

Shepherd, A. (1990). The range of urodynamic investigation. In *Female urinary incontinence* (ed. G. J. Jarvis), pp 21–31. London: Royal College of Obstetricians and Gynaecologists

Takahashi, S., Homma, Y., Fujishiro, T. *et al.* (2000). Electromyographic study of the striated urethral sphincter in type 3 stress incontinence: evidence of myogenic-dominant changes. *Urology* **56**, 946–950.

Toozs-Hobson, P., Athanasiou, S., Khullar, V., Boos, K., Hextall, A. & Cardozo, L. (1997). Does vaginal delivery damage the pelvic floor? *Neurourology and Urodynamics* **16**, 385–386.

Van Waalwijk van Dorn, E. S. C., Remmers, A. & Janknegt, R. A. (1991). Extramural ambulatory urodynamic monitory during natural filling and normal daily activities: evaluation of 100 patients. **146**, 124–131.

Van Waalwijk van Dorn, E. S. C., Remmers, A. & Janknegt, R. A. (1992). Conventional and extramural ambulatory urodynamic testing of the lower urinary tract in female volunteers. *Journal of Urology* **47**, 1319–1326.

Versi, E. (1990). Discriminant analysis of urethral pressure profilometry data for diagnosis of genuine stress incontinence. *British Journal of Obstetrics and Gynaecology* **97**, 251–257.

Versi, E., Cardozo, L. D., Studd, J. W. W. *et al.* (1986). Internal urinary sphincter in the maintenance of female continence. *British Medical Journal* **292**, 166–167.

Versi, E., Orrego, G., Hardy, E. *et al.* (1996). Evaluation of the home pad test in the investigation of female urinary incontinence. *British Journal of Obstetrics and Gynaecology* **103**, 162–167.

Wang, A. C. & Chen, M.-C. (2003). The correlation between preoperative voiding mechanism and surgical outcome of the tension-free vaginal tape procedure with reference to quality of life. *British Journal of Urology International* **91**, 502–506.

Wise, B. G., Burton, G., Cutner, A. & Cardozo, L. D. (1992). Effect of vaginal ultrasound probe on lower urinary tract function. *British Journal of Urology* **70**, 12–16.

PART 3

Evidence and opinion for clinical intervention

Behavioural modifications and physiotherapeutic intervention in stress urinary incontinence

Jeanette Haslam

Introduction

Stress urinary incontinence (SUI) is a major problem in many women's lives. The actual prevalence rate varies between studies, but is generally found to be highest between the ages of 24 and 49 years (Hannestad *et al.* 2000). Although not classed as being life-threatening, SUI is certainly a quality of life issue imposing a significant burden on the women sufferers (Fultz *et al.* 2003). Incontinent women have been found to spend less hours walking, communicating with friends and family by telephone or e-mail, working for pay, using a computer and surprisingly, less time on personal grooming and hygiene than continent women (Fultz *et al.* 2004). Perhaps it is because of embarrassment and the still-present stigma of incontinence that women often delay or never visit their doctor to get help for their problem (Diokno *et al.* 2004; Kinchen *et al.* 2003).

To be continent, a woman not only needs to be neurologically intact, have effective pelvic floor muscles (PFMs) and urethral sphincter mechanism, but also to be mobile and able to access suitable facilities.

There are some factors to be aware of even though they cannot be changed and these include familial predisposition and race. It has been shown that there is an increased familial risk of SUI for a woman if their mother or older sister has SUI (Hannestad *et al.* 2004) and also that Caucasian women are more susceptible to SUI than are Afro-American women (Graham & Mallet 2001) or Black and Hispanic women (Sze *et al.* 2002). Although SUI is predominantly a female condition, men may also suffer from the condition as a consequence of prostatic surgery and basic therapeutic principles of intervention are appropriate; but men are not specifically discussed in this chapter.

It is perhaps necessary to look at the female life events when a therapeutic intervention may be of help and also at the behavioural factors that may be contributory and can be amended before considering the interventions themselves.

Pregnancy and childbirth

There is no doubt that pregnancy and childbirth are associated with SUI. It has also been shown in a follow up study that those women suffering with SUI in pregnancy have twice the risk of suffering SUI 15 years later (Dolan *et al.* 2003). It has been found in a study of 103 women that continent nulliparous pregnant women have statistically significant thicker and stronger PFMs than incontinent nulliparous pregnant women (Morkved *et al.* 2004). It was also previously revealed by the same group of researchers that intensive pelvic floor muscle exercise (PFME) during pregnancy prevents urinary incontinence during pregnancy and in the postpartum ($n = 1$); PFME should therefore be considered as part of preventative care in the antenatal period (Morkved *et al.* 2003). Similarly, Reilly *et al.* (2002) also found that supervised PFME were effective in reducing the risk of postpartum SUI ($n = 268$). More recently, it has also been shown that PFM training in pregnancy resulted in fewer cases of prolonged second stage of labour (Salveson & Morkved 2004).

On reviewing relevant papers of sufficient quality, the Cochrane Group (Hay-Smith *et al.* 2001) found that intensive training was significantly better than standard training for self-reported cure in postnatal women. It can therefore be seen that therapeutic interventions have been successful in pregnancy and the postnatal period without any associated untoward morbidity.

Pelvic surgery and hysterectomy

It has long been debated whether hysterectomy is implicated in pelvic floor dysfunction post surgery. Many studies have taken place with differing results and problems with their methodology (Abdel-Fattah *et al.* 2004). Despite the present lack of evidence, physiotherapists believe that post major gynaecological surgery is an appropriate time to educate women about the PFMs. This involves teaching PFME, the use of a pre-timed contraction as described by Miller *et al.* (1998), posture correction with the use of the transversus abdominis muscles, and correct defaecation techniques. Research is needed to determine if this is a useful or fruitless activity.

The menopause and ageing

The menopause may occur naturally or be accelerated by surgical interventions and women often ascribe their symptoms to starting at the time of the menopause. Atrophic changes that occur at the time of the menopause increase the susceptibility to UTI, this may indeed make women more 'bladder aware'. Although SUI is shown to decrease after the age of 49 there is an increase in mixed urinary symptoms at that time (Hannestad *et al.* 2000). It may be that those women with previous SUI start to have mixed symptoms. However, previous childbirth pelvic floor trauma may not be the major factor at this age as it has been shown that nulliparous, predominantly postmenopausal nuns have similar urinary incontinence prevalence rates as those reported by parous postmenopausal women (Buchsbaum *et al.* 2002). The only relevant factors found were body mass index (BMI), urinary tract infection (UTI) and depression; the use of HRT, hypertension, arthritis, hysterectomy and spinal surgery were not statistically significant (Buchsbaum *et al.* 2002). Another study of 641 women aged 20–59 years found the prevalence of urinary incontinence was increased with age, PFM weakness, genital prolapse, smoking, parity and oestrogen replacement therapy (Samuelsson *et al.* 2000).

Physiotherapists would consider that women of this age group would also benefit from appropriate PFM re-education.

Behavioural modifications

There is a difference in the definition of behavioural therapy in the United Kingdom and in the United States of America. In the UK, the term is generally taken to mean an alteration in lifestyle factors, but in the USA it also encompasses bladder training and pelvic floor therapy. The lifestyle factors that appear to have the most bearing on SUI are obesity, smoking, constipation and strenuous exercise.

Obesity

There have been many reports of an increased BMI being associated with urinary incontinence (Brown *et al.* 1996; Dallosso *et al.* 2003; Elia *et al.* 2001; Rasmussen *et al.* 1997). It has also been shown that weight loss in moderately obese women can improve their incontinence status. Subak *et al.* (2002) studied women with a mean baseline BMI of 38.3 with 13 (±10) incontinence episodes per week. After three months weight reduction, there was great improvement in the frequency of their urinary incontinence. Those women achieving a weight loss of more than 5% had at least a 50% reduction in frequency of incontinence. It would therefore seem appropriate for morbidly and moderately obese women to be offered dietary guidance and advice, especially if they are awaiting surgery.

Smoking

Incontinence has been shown to have an association with people that either smoke or used to smoke more than 20 cigarettes per day (Hannestad *et al.* 2003). This has even been shown in a young population of 18–22 year old women who smoke more than 20 cigarettes a day (Miller *et al.* 2003). It is thought that smokers may have a different mechanism that may cause their incontinence than in non-smokers as they have been found to have stronger urethral sphincters (Bump & McClish 1994). Although smoking cessation is considered good for other health reasons there is no evidence at present that ceasing smoking will resolve problems of incontinence.

Constipation

Women suffering with constipation can inadvertently be affecting their urinary continence status. There are twofold reasons for this: faeces in the rectum can cause pressure on the urethra and bladder neck causing an obstruction to normal micturition and maybe mask SUI, and often repeated straining at stool can cause pudendal nerve damage ultimately resulting in SUI (Bump & Norton 1998). It would therefore seem sensible to ensure that a woman has appropriate dietary advice and be taught defecation technique. However, there do not appear to be any studies that have looked at the effect on continence status of resolving constipation.

Strenuous exercise

It has been shown that urinary incontinence is common in young elite nulliparous athletes (Nygaard et al. 1994). This is not to say that the activities are causing a problem at times other than during the athletic pursuits. It would appear that there is a 'continence threshold' that results in urine loss even when other risk factors are absent. Nygaard et al. (1994) found jumping, high impact landings and running were the most likely to provoke urinary incontinence. However, in a retrospective cohort study, Nygaard (1997) found that participation in high impact activities when young did not result in any higher prevalence rate of clinically significant urinary incontinence when older.

Physiotherapeutic interventions

The Department of Health publication *Good Practice in Continence Services* (Department of Health 2000) states that conservative therapies should be the initial intervention in the management of urinary incontinence in women. A systematic review of randomised clinical trials on the conservative treatment of SUI by Berghmans et al. (1998) found strong evidence to suggest that PFME are an effective therapy in the treatment of SUI. However, the evidence for high-intensity versus low-intensity exercise is limited. Biofeedback was not found to be a more effective adjunct to PFME. Evidence of electrical stimulation effectiveness is clouded by the very many different parameters chosen in different studies. The Cochrane review group (Hay-Smith et al. 2002) concluded that PFM training was better than no treatment or placebo treatment, that intensive exercise was better than standard PFM training and that the effect of adding PFM training to other therapies to the pelvic floor is not clear. Both Berghmans et al. (1998) and Hay-Smith et al. (2002) conclude that further high quality trials are necessary to determine the ultimate therapies.

The following is a description of current physiotherapy practice in the UK.

Assessment

There must be an in-depth history taken and an appropriate physical examination prior to any therapeutic intervention. The history taking should be able to elicit relevant factors from the patient's obstetric, gynaecological, medical and surgical history. Urinalysis should be considered mandatory if there are any symptoms of urgency or frequency. A three-day bladder diary (frequency/volume chart) noting types, volumes and times of fluid taken and times and amounts of urine voided should also be completed by the woman. Ideally, there should be approximately 1500 ml of urine voided per day.

After valid consent (DoH 2001) is given, a physical examination is considered essential. It has been shown by Bø *et al.* (1988) and Bump *et al.* (1991) that verbal and written instructions are insufficient to determine that the woman is able to perform an adequate PFM contraction; some women even bear down believing that they are contracting their PFM. Therefore, to provide only a leaflet or merely describe PFME may be helpful, useless or even harmful.

Before any examination, the relevant anatomy should be discussed, the examination described and instructions given regarding PFM contractions. PFME will underpin any therapeutic intervention for the woman with SUI, it is therefore necessary to carry out a thorough PFM assessment to ensure that any prescribed exercise regimen is possible and appropriate to the individual. It is necessary to examine the abdomen and vagina to determine if there are any other possible contributory factors such as prolapse or constipation. The vaginal examination will also establish if the woman is suitable for other therapies that require instrumentation of the vagina such as the use of vaginal cones, or electrodes.

Details of an appropriate physiotherapy assessment can be found in Laycock (2002).

Pelvic floor muscle exercise

Training of the PFM should be considered initially, as it is an effective, low risk intervention that will contribute towards reducing incontinence significantly (AHCPR 1996). The International Consultation on Incontinence in 2002 cites the exercise science literature of DiNubile (1991) in recommending three sets of eight to 12 slow velocity maximum PFM contractions sustained for 6–8 seconds each, performed three to four times a week for at least 15–20 weeks (Wilson *et al.* 2002). It should not, however, be assumed that this is an appropriate regimen for all women with PFM dysfunction. DiNubile (1991) looked at muscle training from an orthopaedic view regarding athletic performance, not specifically for the needs of individual women with PFM dysfunction following childbirth. He did, however, discuss the need to consider overload and specificity in order to strengthen muscle. That is, muscles need to be overloaded by working harder than normal and exercised in a way that is specific and similar to its normal usage, i.e. functionally.

The vaginal and PFM assessment aims to determine the correct starting point for PFME. The modified Oxford scale (Laycock & Jerwood 2001) is found very useful in clinical practice when examining a woman despite some beliefs that it is not well enough validated. The grading scale is shown in Table 8.1. The modified Oxford scale has been shown to correlate well with surface electromyography and manometry of the PFM (Haslam 1999).

Having determined the grade of PFM activity, the duration of contraction (up to 10 seconds) and repeatability (up to 10 repetitions) is determined, with at least a 4 second rest between each contraction. After a short rest of about one minute the

Table 8.1 The modified Oxford scale for the PFM

Muscle grade	External observation	Internal examination explanation
0	No external indrawing	No activity detected
1	Movement of the perineal	A mere flicker of activity
2	Body observed	A weak contraction without PFM lift
3	An external indrawing	A moderate PFM lift but without resistance
4	Movement of the perineal body can be observed	A good capability to lift PFM against some resistance
5		An ability to lift PFM against more resistance with a strong grip of the examining digit

woman is then asked to attempt one-second maximum holds as quickly and strongly as they can (up to ten contractions). These slow tonic and fast phasic PFMEs form the basis for a bespoke exercise plan for the individual. Progression over the following weeks is made by increasing the length of PFM hold, shortening the rest phase between the contractions and increasing the number of contractions at each exercise session. Submaximal longer contractions may also be practised to assist in achieving change. Women are best advised to exercise in functional positions with concentrated effort three times a day. If requested to exercise too frequently, women often forget and then have a resulting sense of failure. It is best to discuss when suitable times may be for the individual as this varies greatly according to the everyday life of the woman. The main needs are motivation and compliance to the exercise prescription; this is greatly affected by the enthusiasm, realism and knowledge of the physiotherapist.

The purpose of PFM training is to form a better tonic base of the musculature with a greater ability to use the phasic fast fibres when necessary. It has been shown that women who are taught to use a pre-timed PFM contraction prior to occasions of increased intra-abdominal pressure (known as 'the knack') have decreased vesical neck mobility (Miller *et al.* 2001). This will reduce the amount of dorsocaudal displacement and can augment proximal urethral support during stress activity. It is perhaps by practising 'the knack' that reflex activity is encouraged as described by Constantinou & Govan (1982).

It has also been suggested that different body positions with abducted legs can contribute to PFM fitness (Bø 1994). The positions include standing, supine lying, prone lying and prone kneeling.

PFME classes have also become popular both as an initial meeting point to impart information, to give peer group support and to use as group activity sessions. However all patients need to be seen on an individual basis for initial assessment and progress update.

If on examination there is little or no PFM contraction detected by the physiotherapist, other methods have to be employed to elicit activity. The simplest methods involve giving verbal feedback and proprioception. If there are no signs of a PFM contraction or at best only a very weak contraction without any feeling of lift, then neuromuscular electrical stimulation (NMES) is likely to be considered appropriate.

Neuromuscular electrical stimulation

NMES can be used to directly contract the PFM and facilitate cerebral cortex awareness of appropriate activity. This awareness of contraction can be utilised by the woman making a conscious attempt to join in with the stimulated contraction. The aim is one of being able to eventually initiate a PFM contraction herself and be able to participate in a PFME exercise programme. It has been found that voluntary contraction of the PFM is twice as effective as an electrically stimulated contraction at increasing urethral pressure (Bø & Talseth 1997). It has also been shown that a structured programme of PFME is more effective than NMES (Bø *et al.* 1999).

The research-based evidence for NMES is wide with many different parameters being used and authors claiming success. Wilson *et al.* (2002) conclude that there is insufficient evidence to judge if NMES is better than no treatment for women with SUI; further research is necessary to provide proof of worth for a specific regimen. Any clinician deciding to use NMES for SUI must fully understand the rationale behind the different parameters used.

Despite the lack of definitive research evidence for a specific regimen, clinicians still sometimes find that stimulation is necessary for those people in whom other methods of eliciting a PFM contraction have failed. The assessment of the woman should ensure that there are no contra-indications to NMES, these include: an inability to understand the treatment, a lack of valid consent, vaginal infection, known pregnancy, recent haemorrhage in the area, haematoma, vaginal or perineal tissue damage, or malignancy in the area being given active treatment at present. If a woman is devoid of sensation on vaginal assessment it would be inadvisable to commence NMES, but rather refer the woman for further investigations. Any UTI or atrophic vaginitis should be treated before commencing any NMES therapy. A history of sexual abuse should be discussed in a sensitive manner and it is unlikely that stimulation would be appropriate in such a situation.

The recommendation in the UK for comfort and effectiveness is for CE marked equipment to be used that provides a biphasic rectangular pulse with constant current. Parameters that are advocated for SUI are a frequency of 35–40 Hz, 250 μs pulse duration, to produce a forceful contraction whilst minimising any possible adverse affects due to fatigue (Laycock & Vodusek 2002). The duty cycle should be such that the off time is double the on time. The treatment duration is determined on an individual basis, but the clinician is well advised to start with five minutes NMES and monitor any adverse effects and gradually build up the treatment time to 25–30 minutes.

The electrodes that are used must be CE marked, be able to have good contact with the tissues and be used with a water-based gel. If electrodes are for single patient multiple use they must be cleansed and stored appropriately (Barkess-Jones & Haslam 2002).

Magnetic stimulation has also been used in some research studies (Galloway *et al.* 1999; Unsal *et al.* 2003), but at present it is not in common use and there is insufficient robust evidence to prove its value.

Biofeedback

Biofeedback is the utilisation of any of the senses to gain further knowledge of bodily processes. This can be from the feedback given during vaginal assessment by palpation and verbal instructions, to the use of more complicated computerised equipment.

In a systematic review of 24 randomised controlled trials, Berghmans *et al.* (1998) stated that although there were significant effects of biofeedback when tested as an adjunct to PFME, there was no evidence that the addition of biofeedback was any more effective than PFME alone. However, Weatherall (1999) later questioned the statistical methodology used and after a further meta-analysis concluded that biofeedback may be an important adjunct to PFME.

In the UK, biofeedback is used extensively by clinicians to give women a greater insight into their PFM activity and is always associated with an appropriate PFME regimen.

Vaginal palpation can be used to give increased proprioception to ensure that a woman is able to understand as to where she must contract. Putting the PFM on the stretch in a postero-lateral direction during the vaginal assessment can enhance this. Self-examination may also be taught, but it should not be assumed that all women would be happy with this. Prashar *et al.* (2000) found that only 30% of older women were comfortable with touching their own genitalia.

Vaginal cones have also been researched as a method of biofeedback. Plevnik first reported on their use in 1985. In 1988, Peattie and Plevnik (1988) enrolled 39 women into a vaginal cone study. Seventy per cent of the 30 women completing the one-month study reported a subjective improvement. A Cochrane review of all vaginal cone studies by Herbison *et al.* (2001) concluded that vaginal cones are similar in effect to PFMT and NMES, but that larger high quality studies are necessary.

In clinical practice after the appropriate weight of cone is determined (the one that a woman can retain in the vagina whilst walking for one minute), the woman then attempts to retain the cone for increasing lengths of times and increasing levels of

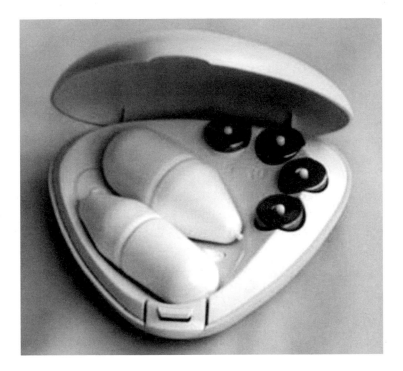

Figure 8.1 Vaginal cones

activity. When she is able to keep a specific weight retained for 15 minutes, the weight of cone is increased and the procedure starts again. Cones can also be used as resistance exercise tools. There are no studies that show cones to be effective as a preventative therapy for incontinence.

The pelvic floor educator was developed from the Periform vaginal electrode in the late 1990s. The body of the indicator is retained within the vagina whilst the wand is external. A downwards deflection of the wand indicates an appropriate PFM contraction, whereas an incorrect valsalva manoeuvre results in an upwards deflection. This tool is utilising similar principles to those espoused by Crystal *et al.* (1971) in the intra-urethral 'Q tip-test'. There is no research base to the use of the educator, however many physiotherapists find it useful in clinical practice.

Manometry has been extensively used as a method of biofeedback. Kegel (1948) was responsible for the earliest vaginal manometers, these have been further developed over many years into sophisticated computerised devices. There can be many problems with manometry, the greatest one being that of ensuring accurate positioning and the maintenance of that position. If the probe is badly positioned in the upper vagina it is likely to be recording intra-abdominal pressure and not that

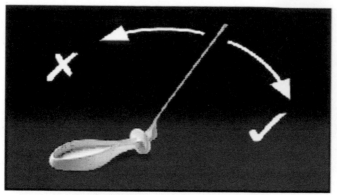

Figure 8.2 The pelvic floor educator

generated by the PFM (Whyte *et al.* 1993). Due to problems with both this and also the use of manometry in functional upright position, it now tends to have been superseded by the use of electromyography (EMG).

Electromyography (EMG) records muscle bioelectrical activity and is a practical indicator of its contractility (Vodusek 1994). The problem with surface EMG is that it is a monitor of and not a measure of activity. Each machine is its own reference and there can be no transferability of outcomes between machines without inter-machine reliability tests being carried out. Electrode placement may also vary, giving different readings. It can therefore be very usefully employed as a further visual and auditory method of giving women further insight into PFM activity but cannot be used to provide outcome measures.

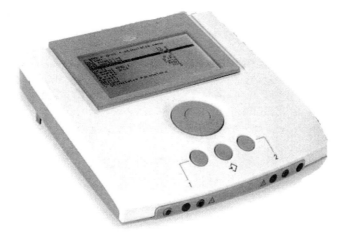

Figure 8.3 Myomed biofeedback equipment

Real time ultrasound is increasingly being used as a tool for biofeedback. It has the advantage of actually visualising PFM activity. At present it has been used extensively as a research tool for recording bladder neck movement during a variety of activities. It has also been used as a tool for teaching PFME (Dietz *et al.* 2001). At present there is no substantial study that shows its effectiveness as a reliable tool for biofeedback therapy for the treatment of SUI.

Other physiotherapy techniques that are also employed have insufficient rigorous research as yet to prove their clinical effectiveness. The main one that physiotherapists have espoused is that of co-contraction of the Transversus abdominis to either reinforce or even activate a PFM contraction. However, the studies so far are all small in number in a largely continent population. However, it does seem likely that research evidence will eventually prove this technique to be beneficial.

It also seems increasingly likely that an assessment of the whole pelvic girdle and its joints may also be essential; any misalignments to be corrected and appropriate exercise espoused. Some physiotherapists also believe that connective tissue mobilisation, Proprioceptive neuromuscular facilitation (PNF), breathing patterns; reflex therapy and acupuncture may all be useful adjuncts to treatment. Again, as yet there is no substantial research-based evidence to show the value of any of these therapies. The next decade should start to unravel some of the mysteries and hopefully provide high quality, research-based evidence regarding effectiveness of further techniques for PFM rehabilitation.

References

Abdel-Fattah, M., Barrington, J., Yousef, M. & Mostafa, A. (2004). Effect of total abdominal hysterectomy on pelvic floor function. *Obstetrical and Gynecological Survey* **59**, 299–304.

Agency for Health Care Policy and Research (AHCPR). *Urinary Incontinence Guideline Panel (1996) Urinary Incontinence in Adults: Acute and Chronic Management*, pp. 36–38. Rockville, Maryland: US Department of Health and Human Services.

Barkess-Jones, L. & Haslam, J. (2002). Infection control issues. In *Therapeutic management of incontinence and pelvic pain* (ed. J. Laycock & J. Haslam), pp. 243–248. London: Springer.

Berghmans, L. C. M., Hendriks, H. J. M., Bø, K., Hay-Smith, E. J., de Bies, R. A., van Waalwijk & van Doorn, E. S. C. (1998). Conservative treatment of stress urinary incontinence in women: a systematic review of randomized clinical trials. *British Journal of Urology* **82**, 181–191.

Bø, K., Larsen, S., Oseid, S., Kvarstein, B., Hagen, R. & Jorgenson, J. (1988). Knowledge about and ability to correct pelvic floor muscle exercises in women with stress urinary incontinence. *Neurourology and Urodynamics* **69**, 261–262.

Bø, K. (1994). Isolated muscle exercises In *Pelvic Floor Re-education. Principles and Practice* (ed. Schüssler, Laycock, Norton & Stanton), pp. 134–138. Berlin: Springer Verlag.

Bø, K. & Talseth, T. (1997). Change in urethral pressure during voluntary pelvic floor muscle contraction and vaginal electrical stimulation. *International Urogynecology Journal and Pelvic Floor Dysfunction* **8**, 3–7.

Bø, K., Talseth, T. & Holme, I. (1999). Single blind, randomised controlled trial of pelvic floor exercises, electrical stimulation, vaginal cones, and no treatment in management of genuine stress incontinence in women. *British Medical Journal* **318**, 487–493.

Brown, J. S., Seeley, D. G., Fong, J., Black, D. M., Ensrud, K.E. & Grady, D. (1996). Urinary incontinence in older women: who is at risk? Study of Osteoporotic Fractures Research Group. *Obstetrics and Gynecology* **87**, 715–721.

Buchsbaum, G. M., Chin, M., Glantz, C. & Guzick, D. (2002). Prevalence of urinary incontinence and associated risk factors in a cohort of nuns. *Obstetrics and Gynecology* **100**, 226-229.

Bump, R. C., Hurt, W. G., Fantl, J. A. & Wyman, J. A. (1991). Assessment of Kegel pelvic muscle exercise performance after brief verbal instruction. *American Journal of Obstetrics and Gynecology* **165**, 322–329.

Bump, R. C. & McClish, D. M. (1994). Cigarette smoking and pure genuine stress incontinence of urine: a comparison of risk factors and determinants between smokers and non smokers. *American Journal of Obstetrics and Gynecology* **170**, 579–582.

Bump, R. C. & Norton, P. A. (1998). Epidemiology and natural history of pelvic floor dysfunction. *Obstetrics and Gynecology Clinics of North America* **25**, 723–746.

Constantinou, C. E. & Govan, D. E. (1982). Spatial distribution and timing of transmitted and reflexly generated urethral pressures in healthy women. *Journal of Urology* **127**, 964–969.

Crystal, D., Charme, L. & Copeland, W. (1971). Q-tip test in stress urinary incontinence. *Obstetrics and Gynecology* **38**, 313–315.

Dallosso, H. M., McGrother, C. W., Matthews, R. J., Donaldson, M. M. & Leicestershire MRC Incontinence Study Group (2003). The association of diet and other lifestyle factors with overactive bladder and stress incontinence: a longitudinal study in women. *BJU International* **92**, 69–77.

Department of Health. (2000). *Good Practice in Continence Services.* London: Department of Health.

Department of Health (2001). *Reference Guide to Consent for Examination or Treatment.* London: Department of Health.

Dietz, H. P., Wilson, P. D. & Clarke, B. (2001). The use of perineal ultrasound to quantify levator activity and teach pelvic floor muscle exercises. *International Urogynecology Journal and Pelvic Floor Dysfunction* **12**, 166–168.

DiNubile, N. A. (1991). Strength training. *Clinics in Sports Medicine* **10**, 33–62.

Diokno, A. C., Burgio, K., Fultz, N. H., Kinchen, K. S., Obenchain, R. & Bump, R. C. (2004). Medical and self-care practices reported by women with urinary incontinence. *American Journal of Managed Care* **10**, 69–78.

Dolan, L. M., Hosker, G. L., Mallett, V. T., Allen, R. E. & Smith, A. R. (2003). Stress incontinence and pelvic floor neurophysiology 15 years after the first delivery. *British Journal of Obstetrics and Gynaecology* **110**, 1107–1114.

Elia, G., Dye, T. D. & Scariati, P. D. (2001). Body mass index and urinary symptoms in women. *International Urogynecology Journal and Pelvic Floor Dysfunction* **12**, 366–369.

Fultz, N. H., Burgio, K, Diokno, A. C., Kinchen, K. S., Obenchain, R. & Bump, R. C. (2003). Burden of stress urinary incontinence for community-dwelling women. *American Journal of Obstetrics and Gynecology* **189**, 1275–1282.

Fultz, N. H., Fisher, G. G. & Jenkins, K. R. (2004). Does urinary incontinence affect middle-aged and older women's time use and activity patterns? *Obstetrics and Gynecology* **104**, 1327–1334.

Galloway, N. T., El-Galley, R. E., Sand, P. K., Appell, R. A., Russell, H. W. & Carlan, S. J. (1999). Extracorporeal magnetic innervation therapy for stress urinary incontinence. *Urology* **53**, 1108–1111.

Graham, C. A. & Mallett, V. T. (2001). Race as a predictor of urinary incontinence and pelvic organ prolapse. *American Journal of Obstetrics and Gynecology* **185**, 116–120.

Hannestad, Y. S., Rortveit, G., Sandvik, H. & Hunskaar, S. (2000). A community based epidemiological survey of female urinary incontinence. The Norwegian EPINCONT study. *Journal of Clinical Epidemiology* **53**, 1150–1157

Hannestad, Y. S., Rortveit, G., Daltveit, A. K. & Hunskaar, S. (2003). Are smoking and other lifestyle factors associated with female urinary incontinence? The Norwegian EPINCONT Study. *British Journal of Obstetrics and Gynaecology* **110**, 247–254.

Hannestad, Y. S., Lie, R. T., Rortveit, G. & Hunskaar, S. (2004). Familial risk of urinary incontinence in women: population based cross sectional study. *British Medical Journal* **329**, 889–891.

Haslam, J. (1999). Evaluation of pelvic floor muscle assessment, digital, manometric and surface electromyography in females. Unpublished MPhil thesis, University of Manchester, UK.

Hay-Smith, E. J. C., Herbison, P. & Morkved, S. (2001). Physical therapy for the prevention of incontinence in adults (Cochrane protocol) 2001. Oxford: Update Software.

Hay-Smith, E. J. C., Bø, K., Berghmans, L. C. M., Hendriks, H. J. M., de Bie, R. A., van Waalwijk, & van Doorn, E. S. C. (2002). Pelvic Floor muscle training for urinary incontinence in women (Cochrane Review). In *The Cochrane Library*, issue 4. Oxford: Update Software.

Herbison, P., Plevnik, S. & Mantle, J. (2001). Weighted vaginal cones for urinary incontinence (Cochrane Review). In *The Cochrane Library*, issue 4, Oxford: Update Software.

Kegel, A. H. (1948). Progressive resistance exercises in the functional restoration of the perineal muscles. *American Journal of Obstetrics and Gynecology* **36**, 238–248.

Kinchen, K. S., Burgio, K., Diokno, A. C., Fultz, N. H., Bump, R. & Obenchain, R. (2003). Factors associated with women's decisions to seek treatment for urinary incontinence. *Journal of Women's Health* **12**, 687–698.

Laycock, J. & Jerwood, D. (2001). Pelvic floor assessment; the PERFECT scheme. *Physiotherapy* **87**, 631–642.

Laycock, J. (2002). Patient assessment. In *Therapeutic management of incontinence and pelvic pain* (ed. J. Laycock & J. Haslam), pp. 45–54. London: Springer.

Laycock, J. & Vodusek, D. B. (2002). Electrical stimulation. In *Therapeutic management of incontinence and pelvic pain* (ed. J. Laycock & J. Haslam), pp. 85–89. London: Springer.

Miller, J. M., Ashton-Miller, J. A. & DeLancey, J. O. L. (1998). A pelvic muscle pre-contraction can reduce cough related urine loss in selected women with mild SUI. *Journal of the American Geriatric Society* **46**, 870–874.

Miller, J. M., Perucchini, D, Carchidi, L.T., DeLancey, J. O. & Ashton-Miller, J. (2001). Pelvic floor muscle contraction during a cough and decreased vesical neck mobility. *Obstetrics and Gynecology* **97**, 255–260.

Miller, Y. D., Brown, W. J., Russell, A. & Chiarelli, P. (2003). Urinary incontinence across the lifespan. *Neurourology and Urodynamics* **22**, 550–557.

Morkved, S., Bø, K., Schei, B. & Salveson, K. A. (2003). Pelvic floor muscle training during pregnancy to prevent urinary incontinence: a single-blind randomized controlled trial. *Obstetrics and Gynecology* **101**, 313–319.

Morkved, S., Salvesen, K. A., Bø, K. & Eik-Nes, S. (2004). Pelvic floor muscle strength and thickness in continent and incontinent nulliparous pregnant women. *International Urogynecology Journal and Pelvic Floor Dysfunction* **15**, 384–390.

Nygaard, I. E., Thompson, F. L., Svengalis, S. L. & Albright, J. P. (1994). Urinary incontinence in elite nulliparous athletes. *Obstetrics and Gynecology* **84**, 183–187.

Nygaard, I. E. (1997). Does prolonged high-impact activity contribute to later urinary incontinence? A retrospective cohort study of female Olympians. *Obstetrics and Gynecology* **90**, 718–722.

Plevnic, S. (1985). New method for testing and strengthening of pelvic floor muscles. In *Proceedings of the 15th Annual Meeting, International Continence Society*, pp. 267–268.

Peattie, A. B. & Plevnik, S. (1988). Vaginal cones: a conservative method of treating genuine stress incontinence. *British Journal of Obstetrics and Gynaecology* **95**, 1049–1053.

Prashar, S., Simons, A., Bryant, C., Dowell, C. & Moore, K. H. (2000). Attitudes to vaginal/urethral touching and device placement in women with urinary incontinence. *International Urogynecology Journal and Pelvic Floor Dysfunction* **11**, 4–8.

Rasmussen, K. L., Krue, S., Johansson, L. E., Knudsen, H. J. & Agger, A. O. (1997). Obesity as a predictor of postpartum urinary symptoms. *Acta Obstetricia et Gynecologica Scandinavica* **76**, 359–362.

Reilly, E. T., Freeman, R. M., Waterfield, M. R., Waterfield, A. E., Steggles, P. & Pedlar, F. (2002). Prevention of postpartum stress incontinence in primigravidae with increased bladder neck mobility: a randomised controlled trial of antenatal pelvic floor exercises. *British Journal of Obstetrics and Gynaecology* **109**, 68–76.

Salvesen, K. A. & Morkved, S. (2004). Randomised controlled trial of pelvic floor muscle training during pregnancy. *British Medical Journal* **14**, 378–380.

Samuelsson, E., Victor, A. & Svardsudd, K. (2000). Determinants of urinary incontinence in a population of young and middle-aged women. *Acta Obstetricia et Gynecologica Scandinavica* **79**, 208–215.

Subak, L. L., Johnson, C., Whitcomb, E., Boban, D., Saxton, J. & Brown, J.S. (2002). Does weight loss improve incontinence in moderately obese women? *International Urogynecology Journal and Pelvic Floor Dysfunction* **13**, 40–43.

Sze, E. H., Jones, W. P., Ferguson, J. L., Barker, C. D. & Dolezal, J. M. (2002). Prevalence of urinary incontinence symptoms among black, white, and Hispanic women. *Obstetrics and Gynecology* **99**, 572–575.

Unsal, A., Saglam, R. & Cimentepe, E. (2003). Extracorporeal magnetic stimulation for the treatment of stress and urge incontinence in women—results of 1-year follow-up. *Scandinavian Journal of Urology and Nephrology* **37**, 424–428.

Vodusek, D. (1994). Electrophysiology. In *Pelvic Floor Re-education* (ed. B. Schussler, J. Laycock, P. Norton & S. Stanton), pp. 83–97. London: Springer.

Weatherall, M. (1999). Biofeedback or pelvic floor muscle exercises for female genuine stress incontinence: a meta-analysis of trials identified in a systematic review. *BJU International* **83**, 1015–1016.

Whyte, T. D., McNally, D.S. & James, E. D. (1993). Six-element sensor for measuring vaginal pressure profiles. *Medical and Biological Engineering and Computing* **31**, 184–186

Wilson, P. D., Bø, K., Hay-Smith, J., Nygaard, I., Staskin, D., Wyman, J. & Bourcier, A. (2002). Conservative treatment in women. In *Incontinence*, second edition (ed. P. Abrams, L. Cardozo, S. Khoury & A. Wein), pp. 573–624. London: Health Publication.

Chapter 9

Containment and stress urinary incontinence: current perspectives in product provision, usage and evaluation

Mandy Fader, Donna Zimmaro Bliss, Sinead Clarke-O'Neill, Alan Cottenden, Kathyrn Getliffe, Hector H. Herrera, Jan Paterson, George Szonyi and Mary Wilde

Introduction

Products for stress urinary incontinence (SUI) provide an alternative to surgery, and latterly medication, for a large number of women. The type of products available may be broadly split into two categories: absorbent products and occlusive devices.

Absorbent products are available in a wide range of different designs and absorbencies and may be washable or disposable. They suit very light incontinence through to the heavier end of light/moderate incontinence. There have been relatively few studies of these products and those that have been conducted have a tendency to quickly become out of date as products are frequently discontinued and new products introduced. However, it is possible to draw some broad conclusions from the studies to guide practice.

Female occlusive devices are very varied in design and although many have been introduced to the market, few of these products are still available. They may be subdivided into three categories: those that occlude at the external meatus, those that occlude in the urethra (intraurethral devices) or those that occlude via the vagina (intravaginal devices). These products do not suit all women with SUI and their efficacy is marred by poor acceptability. However, there is clearly a place for these devices in management as they do perform effectively for some women, and evaluations of these products have provided some promising results. Unfortunately, because of the small market, many of the devices are no longer commercially available, so those who may have benefited are denied the opportunity to try them. This chapter reviews the research evidence examining the efficacy of absorbent and occlusive products for women with SUI.

Absorbent products for women with light incontinence

Absorbent products are designed to absorb urine and then to be either thrown away or washed and reused. There are four main product designs for women with light incontinence:

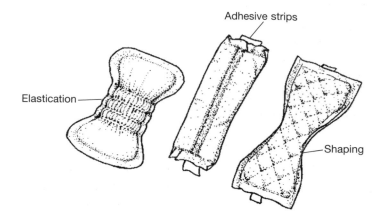

Figure 9.1 Disposable insert pads

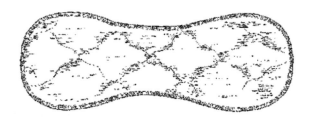

Figure 9.2 Washable insert pad

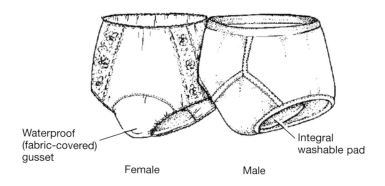

Figure 9.3 Washable pants with integral pad

- Disposable inserts (Figure 9.1)
- Washable inserts (Figure 9.2)
- Disposable pull-up pants with integral pad
- Washable pants with integral pad (Figure 9.3)

The disposable pull-up group are relatively expensive, single-use items and are seldom used for light incontinence except as 'special occasion' items. Underpads are not commonly used for light incontinence.

Evaluation, quality of data and results

A small number of robust comparative evaluations of absorbent pads for lightly incontinent women have been published (Table 9.1). One study has compared a range of disposable inserts and menstrual pads and there have been comprehensive single group studies of disposable inserts and washable pants with integral pads. There have been no published studies of reusable inserts for light incontinence. Nor have there been any studies directly comparing different design groups to determine which designs are most effective and no cost-effectiveness data have been published. However, taking all these studies together, it is possible to draw cautious broad conclusions about the effectiveness of different product designs. A further study has compared specially made experimental products that have differed from one another in carefully controlled ways enabling more specific questions about product materials and design to be addressed.

Table 9.1 Studies evaluating absorbent products for women with light incontinence

Product name/design	Author	Number of subjects
Disposable inserts	Clarke-O'Neill et al. (2004)	60
Disposable inserts	Thornburn et al. (1997)	20
Disposable inserts and sanitary towels	Baker & Norton (1996)	65
Washable pants with integral pad	Clarke-O'Neill et al. (2002)	72

Using a multiple crossover design, Clarke-O'Neill et al. (2004) compared the range (12 products) of disposable inserts for lightly incontinent women available in the UK in 2000. Products were tested by 60 community-based women aged 50 years or older who currently used products similar to those to be evaluated. Products were evaluated using a pad-performance questionnaire and a pad-leakage diary. As a group, the products performed well in terms of their ability to hold urine without leakage. Pad-leakage diary results from 5761 saved pads showed that although the mode urine weight was 8 g, the range was wide (0–180 g). The frequency distribution showed a long tail with around a third of pads having a urine weight of more than 40 g. The best-performing product showed a leakage performance of 95% (CI 81–99%) of pads not leaking at all with 10 g of urine and 92% (CI 78–98%) with 20 g of urine. By comparison, 81% (CI 67–89%) of the worst-performing product did not leak at all with 10 g of urine and 76% (CI 63–86%) with 20 g of urine. However, the 'overall opinion' scores of the testers showed much greater differences between products with 88% of subjects scoring the most successful insert as Good or OK compared with 51% for the least successful product ($p < 0.001$) (Level of Evidence 2).

A similar study by the same research group (Clarke-O'Neill *et al.* 2002) compared all the ten reusable pants with integral pad for lightly incontinent women available in the UK in 1999. Seventy-two community-based women who usually used absorbent products for light incontinence tested each product for 1 week each. Leakage performance was found to be disappointing with 69% (CI 59–78%) of the best-performing product not leaking at all with 10 g of urine, compared with 40% (CI 29–51%) for the least successful product. Again, subjects' 'overall opinion' scores showed wide differences with the best-performing product scoring 85% Good or OK compared with 34% for the least successful product (Level of Evidence 2).

A comparison between the results of these two studies (Table 9.2) shows that, for community-based women with light incontinence, disposable insert pads are more effective at preventing leakage than reusable pants with integral pad, but the best products in the two groups had similar scores for 'overall opinion'.

Table 9.2 Comparison between findings from two studies: (1) disposable inserts (2) washable pants with integral pad (Clarke-O'Neill *et al* 2004; Clarke-O'Neill *et al* 2002)

	Most successful disposable insert	Most successful reusable pants with integral pad
Overall opinion:		
Good	57%	58%
OK	31%	27%
Poor	12%	15%
Per cent of pads not leaking at all for:		
10 g of urine	96% (CI 86–99)	69% (CI 59–78)
20 g of urine	89% (CI 76–95)	44% (CI 32–57)

However, comparisons between these data must be made cautiously because these were two separate studies undertaken with two different, albeit similar, populations. It is likely that reusable pants are cheaper in the long-term than disposable inserts, assuming that they have a reasonably long life (in excess of 50 washes), but economic comparisons have not been studied. Reusable pants have a more 'normal' appearance than disposable inserts and are likely to be particularly useful for occasional incontinence when often disposable pads would still be dry when discarded.

Baker and Norton (1996) evaluated six small disposable inserts and two sanitary towels (available in the USA in 1991) with 65 community-dwelling women. The products were rated using an evaluation questionnaire and daily diary of pad use. The two menstrual pads (which were the least expensive pads in the study) scored significantly higher than many of the incontinence products, although neither was the most popular pad. The authors concluded that women should try a 'maxi' menstrual pad first and then move onto a higher capacity (incontinence) pad if this is inadequate. However, products have changed considerably since this study was carried out and the current relative performance of menstrual pads compared with disposable inserts for incontinence is not known (Level of Evidence 2).

Thornburn *et al.* (1997) compared three variants of a small, shaped disposable pad by asking 20 lightly incontinent women living in the community (age range 37–89 years) to evaluate each in turn for a week in random order. Women then blind tested a random sequence of 42 pads (14 of each variant) scoring the performance of each individual pad. One variant was engineered to have high absorbency and good wetback (resistance to allowing fluid to escape back on to the wearer's skin) by using a hydrophobic coverstock and including a substantial quantity of superabsorber in the core. A second variant had a hydrophilic coverstock and no superabsorber, chosen to give low absorbency and poor wetback. The third variant had intermediate properties. Whenever differences in wet comfort, absorbency or overall performance were found they were in the expected order, but differences were small and few reached statistical significance. The clinical value of including technically superior materials was not strongly supported. However, this was a small study and may have had insufficient power to detect significant differences (Level of Evidence 2).

Summary

As a design group, disposable inserts are more effective at containing leakage than reusable pants with integral pad (Level of Evidence 3). However, the individual products within both design groups exhibit a wide range of performance and acceptability for individuals, and it cannot therefore be assumed that a single brand of product will be as acceptable or effective in terms of leakage performance as another (Level of Evidence 2). Some reusable pants with integral pad were well-liked by patients and may be an acceptable alternative to disposable inserts for those who prefer a more 'normal' appearance or for women with very light incontinence (Level of Evidence 3). Menstrual pads may be as effective as some disposable inserts (Level of Evidence 3).

- Absorbent products are the mainstay of continence management for SUI.
- Disposable inserts are good for leakage, and have a high acceptability rating.
- Washable pants perform relatively poorly for leakage, but have a high acceptability rating.

Recommendations

Most disposable inserts for light incontinence are likely to be satisfactory for patients in terms of leakage, but patients may have individual preferences and should be offered a selection to try where possible (Grade of Recommendation B). Sanitary towels may be sufficient for some patients with very light incontinence (Grade of Recommendation C). Reusable pants are an acceptable and probably cost-effective alternative to disposable inserts for women with very light incontinence, but are more likely to leak than disposable inserts and are not recommended for heavier urine loss (Grade of Recommendation B).

Priorities for research

Reusable pants need to be compared directly with disposable inserts and current menstrual pads, including an economic analysis.

Female occlusive devices: devices that occlude at the external meatus

Urethral occlusion devices have been developed to block urinary leakage at the external urethral meatus. Several devices have utilised either adhesive or mild suction to occlude urinary loss at the urethral meatus. In addition to the simple barrier effect, compression of the wall of the distal urethra has been hypothesised to contribute to continence. There are three brands, two of which are no longer marketed:

- Miniguard (Uromed, *no longer available*)
- FemAssist (Insight Medical, *no longer available*)
- Capsure (Bard, *USA only*)

Miniguard is an angular-shaped foam device that utilises an adhesive hydrogel to adhere to the peri-meatal area. The device is single use, removed prior to voiding, and disposable. FemAssist (Figure 9.4), is a small hat-shaped silicone device that adheres by applying an adhesive gel to the edge of the device, squeezing the central dome and creating a vacuum. The device is then placed over the urethral meatus and, upon release, the meatal mucosa is drawn up into the device and the urethral lumen is occluded. It may be worn for up to 4 hours or until voiding, after which the device is washed in hot soapy water and reapplied. The device is reusable for 1 week. CapSure is applied and retained by suction. A petroleum-based lubricant is applied before device use. The device is removed for voiding and re-utilised for up to 2 weeks.

Evaluation, quality of data and results

There have been no randomised controlled trials of these products, study designs have been open and longitudinal and have lasted between 4 weeks and 3 months. There have been no recent studies of these products and the majority of the studies were

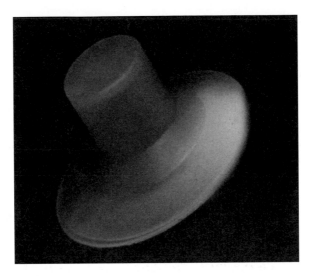

Figure 9.4 FemAssist

carried out in the late 1990s. Urinary diaries and pad-weight tests were employed in all studies for objective efficacy measurements on Miniguard, FemAssist and CapSure. Incontinence impact questionnaires (IIQ), visual analogue score (VAS), quality of life (QoL) and/or urogenital distress inventory (UDI) were also used. (Table 9.3).

Table 9.3 Studies evaluating external urethral occlusive devices

Device name	Author	Number of subjects
Miniguard	Eckford *et al.* (1996)	19
	Brubaker *et al.* (1999)	390
FemAssist	Versi & Harvey (1998)	133
	Moore et al. (1999b)	57
	Tincello *et al.* (1997)	27
	Tincello *et al.* (2000)	41
Capsure	Bellin *et al.* (1998)	88
	Shinopulos *et al.* (1999)	84

Miniguard

A study by Eckford *et al.* (1996) looked at the efficacy of a single application of this device during a 1-h pad test and reported that 25% of patients were continent, 50% were improved, but 25% had worse incontinence. In a large study by Brubaker *et al.* (1999), 648 women were recruited for a study of whom 411 enrolled, 390 used the device and 346 completed the study. Of the 65 who enrolled but did not start the trial,

21 withdrew before device use, 17 were lost to follow-up, 12 withdrew for device-related reasons and there were 6 protocol violations. Symptoms of vulvar irritation or lower urinary tract discomfort occurred in a small percentage of subjects but were generally transient and only 3 women discontinued using the device for this reason. Also noted was a persistence of efficacy ($p < 0.001$) 4 weeks following device discontinuation (Level of Evidence 3).

FemAssist

Versi & Harvey (1998) studied 155 women with stress or mixed incontinence, of whom 133 attempted to use FemAssist and 96 enrolled in a 4-week study. Their mean pad-test loss fell from 27 to 9.4 g ($p < 0.001$) and 49% were dry. Symptomatic cure was more likely in those with mild incontinence. Of the 9 women who had a positive pad test (> 2 g) without the device, 5 were dry (< 2 g) with the device ($p < 0.05$). VAS scores showed a significant improvement for the symptom of stress incontinence ($p < 0.05$). QoL scores improved significantly by 38% ($p < 0.05$) for the IIQ and 29% ($p < 0.0$ 1) for UDI (Level of Evidence 3).

Moore *et al.* (1999b) reported on 57/100 recruited women who completed a 1-month trial. Reduction of incontinence was statistically significant for pad testing, which revealed that 47% of the patients became continent and 33% had more than 50% benefit compared with baseline, while 9% had worse leakage. Those with severe baseline leakage were equally likely to respond as those with mild or moderate pad-test loss. Women with stress urge or mixed incontinence appeared to respond equally well. Dropouts included 13% who were unwilling to utilise the device (Level of Evidence 3).

Tincello *et al.* (1997) carried out a 3-month prospective study involving 27 women with urodynamic stress incontinence. They found the median (range) loss with and without the device was 4.9 (0–65) and 21 (1–94) ml, respectively ($p < 0.01$), and 20 patients were less wet when using the device. Discomfort was greater among the women with a greater loss. The acceptability correlated negatively with discomfort ($r = -0.53$) and negatively with embarrassment ($r = -0.39$); 15 patients (56%) reported that they would use the device in the long-term (Level of Evidence 3). Tincello *et al.* (2000) later reported on 41 women recruited to use the device over a 3-month period, but 10 declined to participate, 6 withdrew before 2 weeks, 10 failed to attend the 2-week follow-up and 11 did not attend the 3-month follow-up. Only 2 completed the study. There was no difference in pad-test or voiding-diary grades. The authors concluded that the device had low acceptability and was ineffective, and could not be recommended for non-surgical management of stress incontinence (Level of Evidence 3).

CapSure

Bellin *et al.* (1998) reported on 88/100 completers after 12 weeks, with 82% elimination of leakage on pad test, 91% continent on provocative stress test (single cough assessment of leakage) and 48% dry and 40% improved on urinary diaries. Pad-test leakage decreased from 6.67 (range 0.55–25.95) to 0.19 g (range 0–2.5) by week 12. Five patients withdrew secondary to vaginal irritation and 3 due to poor device fit (Level of Evidence 3).

Shinopulos *et al.* (1999) carried out a multicentre study enrolling 100 women with stress incontinence who wore the device for 12 weeks; 84 women completed the study. Mean pad weights reduced from 6.7 g at baseline to 0.19 g by week 12. Complications affected 7 patients including urethral/vaginal swelling and vulval abrasion, but none of the affected patients withdrew from the study. The quality of life (I-QoL) tool showed significant mean improvement from 62.3 to 90.4.

Summary

External urethral occlusive devices were found to be of varying efficacy, with minimal morbidity. Efficacy of the combined studies reveals a continence rate of approximately 50% dry and 2/3 of patients improved. Devices achieve occlusion either by blocking at the meatus or compressing the distal urethral lumen, and adherence to the peri-meatal area is essential to success. However, the method and degree of adherence is also the determining factor for the type and severity of local irritation. Patient selection based on motivation, appropriate anatomy and manual dexterity, in combination with efficacy and morbidity, will determine overall satisfaction. There are no data which compare one extraurethral device to another, or to other categories of products. Cost comparisons for disposable versus short-term reusable devices are not available. Efficacy for different grades of incontinence has not been established. The objective degree of continence improvement in the clinical laboratory (pad and stress tests) is greater than in community use (diaries).

- Combined studies show a continence rate of approximately 50% dry and 2/3 improved.
- Local irritation is a common side effect.
- There are no randomised controlled trials comparing different external devices or comparing other categories of products.
- The products have failed to find popularity with users and clinicians.
- The products are not commercially available in the UK.

Priorities for research

Further research on the development and role of devices which block urinary leakage at the external urinary meatus, with a focus on improving patient acceptability, is recommended. One half of patients utilising these devices in monitored studies were dry and 2/3 of the patients were improved with minimal morbidity. These devices may have a future role in the algorithm of conservative treatment based on patient acceptance, availability and cost, especially in those patients with mild or moderate stress incontinence who prefer to avoid pads or surgery.

Female occlusive devices: intraurethral devices

Urethral inserts are silicone cylinders that are self-inserted or removed at the patient's discretion. They are intended for daytime use, especially during vigorous physical exercise. While some women manage exercise incontinence by limiting fluid intake before or during exercise, by choosing sports that allow frequent bathroom access or wearing absorbent pads, 20–40% of women cope with leakage by ceasing exercise (Dunn *et al.* 2002b). These devices present external retainers or flanges to prevent intravesical migration and proximal balloons to hold the device in place. They act by causing occlusion either in the urethra itself or at the external urethral meatus (Balmforth & Cardozo 2003). There are three brands, two of which are no longer marketed:

- FemSoft (Rochester Medical)
- Viva (*no longer available*)
- Reliance (Uromed, *no longer available)*

The FemSoft (Rochester Medical), shown alongside the Reliance in Figure 9.5 below, is the only urethral insert currently distributed. It has a soft, compressible, mineral oil-filled silicone layer with an insertion probe. Before insertion, the fluid distends the proximal end of the cylinder. As the user pushes the device (guided by the insertion probe) into the urethra, fluid transfers automatically to the distal end, allowing the device to pass through the urethra. Once in place, fluid flows back to the proximal end to hold the device in place. None of these devices are recommended for reuse after removal. The FemSoft Insert is currently packaged in a box of 28 inserts and each box is priced at £27.76 ($49.95). The Viva (Nielsen *et al.* 1993) and Reliance devices are not currently available on the market.

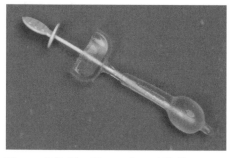
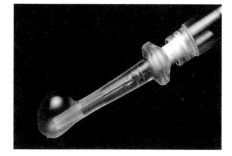

Figure 9.5 The Femsoft and Reliance

Evaluation, quality of data and results

There have been no randomised controlled trials of these devices, and studies that have been conducted have used objective efficacy measurements including the 1-h pad test, voiding diary and QoL questionnaires (Table 9.4).

Table 9.4 Studies evaluating intraurethral occlusive devices

Device name	Authors	Number of subjects
Viva	Peschers *et al.* (1996)	21
	Nielsen *et al.* (1993)	40
Reliance	Staskin *et al.* (1996)	135
	Sand *et al.* (1999)	63
	Miller & Bavendam (1996)	63
Reliance versus FemAssist	Boos *et al.* (1998)	102
FemSoft	Dunn *et al.* (2002b)	6
	Tincello *et al.* (2000)	41

Nielsen *et al.* (1993) and Peschers *et al.* (1996) studied the Viva device. Peschers *et al.* screened 53 patients with SUI and 21 patients accepted treatment with the two-sphere device. During a 4-month study, the investigators analysed subjective improvement and performed pad-weight and cough tests. Nielsen *et al.* demonstrated 94% improvement on leakage and Peschers *et al.* 67% improvement.

Staskin *et al.* (1996) reported on a 4-month study of 135 of 215 patients who utilised a disposable balloon-tipped urethral insert made from thermoplastic elastomer, inflated with an applicator on insertion and deflated by pulling a string at the meatal plate for removal during voiding (Reliance). Eighty subjects discontinued the device early, the main reasons being discomfort and inability or unwillingness to use the device. Of those that continued with the device and 72% reported complete dryness, while 17% showed improvement, from diary data. Pad-test data showed 80% complete dryness and 15% improvement.

Miller & Bavendam (1996) and Sand *et al.* (1999) then reported on 63 of the 135 patients from the above cohort who utilised the device for 1 year. Miller & Bavendam reported 79% complete dryness and 16% significant improvement from pad-weight data, which was also consistent with the improvement in subjective diaries ($p < 0.0001$). The patients reported improved comfort and ease of use over time, with sensation of device presence decreasing from 35% at week 1 to 7% at 12 months. The volume of urine lost during exercise decreased from a median of 20 g (range 4.9–80.2 g) without the insert to 2.6 g (1.3–6.8 g) when the insert was worn ($p = 0.03$). On a 5-point scale in which 1 represented very comfortable and 5 very uncomfortable, subjects rated the mean comfort for the sessions performed with the insert in place as 2.1.

Treatment for positive urine cultures was undertaken in 20% of symptomatic and 11% of asymptomatic patients, 39% of patients had positive cultures which were not treated and 30% had negative cultures at all monthly intervals for the 4-month study. One or more episodes of gross haematuria (24%), cystoscopic findings of mucosal irritation at 4 or at 12 months (9%) and asymptomatic bacteriuria (30%) on monthly cultures were also documented (Miller & Bavendam 1996).

Recent studies have investigated the efficacy of the FemSoft, the only device available. Dunn *et al.* (2002b) measured pad weights during four standardised aerobics sessions during which six subjects were randomly assigned to exercise twice with the insert and without it. The medians of the averaged pad weights for the two different types of sessions were compared. Median urine loss during standardised exercise sessions decreased from 20 g (range 4.9–80.2 g) without the device to 2.6 g (range 1.3–6.8 g) with the device ($p = 0.03$). Five women used the device at home during unsupervised exercise, and one subject had urinary tract infection. At the end of 3 months, satisfaction and comfort were rated high on a 5-point scale. The conclusion was that the FemSoft urethral device is an effective, safe and comfortable treatment for exercise incontinence in women (Level of Evidence 3).

Results from a prospective 3-year study Food and Drug Administration (FDA) post-approval device safety study submitted by Rochester Medical, 2002 unpublished) for evaluation of the long-term effect of the device involved 41 subjects. Of the group, 9 women were 65 years or older (22%, 9/41); 80% were post-menopausal with 24 women (59%) being on hormone replacement. Thirty-eight (93%) used absorbent products to contain urine leakage prior to enrolment. A total of 66 follow-up visits took place with an average participation period of 4.2 years. Seven patients withdrew in the third year, three due to non-study-related health problems and one because of dissatisfaction due to urge symptoms. Two were lost to follow-up. There was a significant difference in the rates of incontinence at the 3-year follow-up between users and non-users of the device: 0.83 versus 2.64 episodes per day, according to voiding diaries. The difference in urine loss during pad-weighing tests was also significant. There were 24 reported adverse events in the 41 subjects enrolled. None of these events required medical intervention except for antibiotic prescription in cases of urinary tract infection. The 24 events included: bacteriuria (11); symptomatic urinary tract infection (3); urinary symptoms (3); device-performance problems (2); irritation (2); and migration (1).

In 33 women a total of 38 cystoscopies were performed at 3 years. Only 1 patient was reported to have an abnormal finding, but this was due to mucosal irritation produced by an indwelling Foley catheter during one hospitalisation for a problem unrelated to the device. Patient satisfaction had not changed over the follow-up time interval. The QoL questionnaire (I-QoL) scores at 3 years were compared with those at 12 months and there was improvement from the baseline of 60.6 to 74.0. No safety concerns concerning urethral integrity were identified after the 3 years of continuous use. The incidence of urinary tract infections, given the high number of insertions and removals, was considered low risk (Level of Evidence 3).

Intraurethral versus external meatus devices

Boos *et al.* (1998) reported in an abstract, a randomised prospective parallel group trial comparing the Reliance intraurethral insert with the FemAssist external meatal occlusive device. Assessments at baseline, 1 month, and 3 months included subjective efficacy, 7-day diary and pad test (1-h). Fifty-three women were randomised to FemAssist and 49 to Reliance device. There were some initial problems with sizing the Reliance. Once this was corrected, 40.8% (20) of women were subjectively dry and the remainder improved on completing the trial. Of women using the FemAssist, 28.3% (15) were dry, 60.4% (32) were improved, 9.4% (5) were no better and only 1 subject was made worse with device use. Problems experienced were few and minor with no serious adverse events. The conclusion was that both devices are efficacious, the FemAssist was more comfortable, but required a greater degree of user skill to achieve control of leakage (Level of Evidence 2).

Summary

Intraurethral devices have demonstrated high efficacy, but have been associated with urinary tract infection, haematuria and discomfort. Bacteriuria, without symptomatic infection, was similar to extraurethral device use, which approaches screening urinalysis data (Brubaker *et al.* 1999), or may be similar to the rates seen with self-catheterisation. Device migration into the bladder, which requires endoscopic removal, is the most serious reported problem. Long-term results are limited. Patient and physician acceptance of this form of therapy has also been limited. The patient needs to have good hand dexterity in order to use these devices and the cost is also a factor that precludes more widespread use (Level of Evidence 3).

- Intraurethral devices appear to have high efficacy, but are associated with urinary tract infection, haematuria and discomfort.
- Device migration is the most serious reported problem.
- Good hand dexterity is needed.
- Cost is high.
- Patient and physician acceptance is limited.
- May be most appropriate for intermittent and occasional use (for example, during exercise).

Recommendations

Intraurethral occlusive devices may be considered for women with stress incontinence but they are invasive devices with high cost and have had limited evaluation. They may be most appropriate for intermittent and occasional use (such as during vigorous exercise) (Grade of Recommendation C).

Priorities for research

It is important that new devices, and in particular invasive ones, be evaluated by randomised trials and compared with approved control devices. Long-term follow-up results are needed to demonstrate the effects of such devices on the urethra and/or bladder and will determine the real value and safety of devices that initially have been adopted enthusiastically.

Further development and study of the use of intraurethral devices for the treatment of urinary incontinence is recommended. The role of intraurethral devices in patients who do not achieve the desired efficacy with other forms of conservative therapy, and to avoid surgery, requires further study.

Intravaginal devices

Support of the bladder neck to correct urinary stress incontinence has been achieved, with varying success, utilising three main approaches: (1) tampons, (2) pessaries and contraceptive diaphragms, and (3) intravaginal devices specifically designed to support the bladder neck (Figure 9.6). Intravaginal devices comprise:

- Tampons
- Pessaries
- Intravaginal ring (Introl, Contiform)
- Disposable foam device (Contrelle Activguard)
- Polyvinyl alcohol sponge (Ladycon)

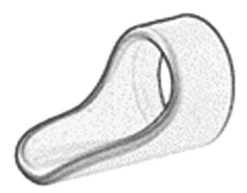

Figure 9.6 Diagrammatic illustration of an intravaginal device

Evaluation quality of data and results (Table 9.5)

Tampons/pessaries

Nygaard (1995) performed a prospective, randomised, single-blind and laboratory-based study testing 18 patients (aged 33–73 years) with three 40-min standardised aerobics sessions, utilising a Hodge pessary, a super tampon or no device. Urine loss was determined by a change in the weight of the pad worn while exercising. Statistical analysis of the log of urine loss revealed that women lost significantly less urine when exercising with either the pessary or the tampon than when exercising with no device. Continence rates were 6/14 cured and 2/14 improved with tampons, and 4/10 improved with a pessary (Level of Evidence 2).

Table 9.5 Studies evaluating intravaginal devices

Device name	Authors	Number of subjects
Tampon/pessary	Nygaard (1995)	18
Diaphragms/pessaries	Realini & Walters (1990)	10
	Suarez *et al.* (1991)	12
	Bhatia & Bergman (1985)	102
Introl	Biswas (1988)	Pilot
	Davila (1996)	53
	Moore *et al.* (1999a)	80
	Moore *et al.* (1999b)	21
	Kondo *et al.* (1997)	57
Continence Guard	Thyssen & Lose (1996)	26
	Thyssen *et al.* (1999)	19
	Sander *et al.* (1999)	55
	Hahn & Milsom (1996)	121
Conveen Continence Guard versus Conveen Continence Tampon	Thyssen *et al.* (2001)	94
Polyvinyl sponge (Ladycon)	Glavind (1997)	6

Diaphragms/pessaries

Realini & Walters (1990) analysed the benefit for 1 week, in 10 selected patients of a coil-type diaphragm ring, which was softer than a pessary, utilising diaries and a 2-h pad test. They also gave an overall subjective evaluation of their experience. Urodynamic findings were essentially unchanged by wearing diaphragm rings. Four of the 10 women experienced clinically significant improvement in amount of urine lost during pad tests, number of leaks per week and overall assessment response (Level of Evidence 3).

Suarez *et al.* (1991) included urodynamic testing in his evaluation of a contraceptive diaphragm in 12 patients. Complete resolution of SUI was achieved in 11 of 12 patients (91%); 2 of the 12 achieved continence but withdrew from the study because of associated discomfort from the diaphragm, therefore, complete resolution of SUI was achieved in 9/12 patients (75%) (Level of Evidence 3).

Bhatia & Bergman (1985) reported on the urodynamic effects of the Hodge pessary on 30 women aged 29–71 years with a history of urinary incontinence. With the pessary, 24 of the 30 patients became continent when tested in the supine position with a full bladder, 3 of the 24 patients lost urine with coughing in the standing position and demonstrated a positive cough profile despite the presence of the vaginal pessary. Uroflowmetry data show that the vaginal pessary did not produce any obstruction to the free flow of urine and suggested this is a modality to predict the outcome for bladder neck support surgery.

Intravaginal devices designed specifically to support the bladder neck:

Included in this category are:

- Removable reusable intravaginal ring, composed of silastic, and constructed with two prongs that are placed behind the symphysis to support the bladder neck (Introl, *no current distributor*).
- Three different single-use disposable devices:
- 1. A clam-type device composed of polyurethane foam that is folded up upon its long axis and placed into the sagittal plane in the vagina. When moistened its dimensions expand by 30% and create a supportive cushion under the urethrovesical junction (previously known as Continence Guard; now available as Contrelle Activgard, Codan Gmbh).
- 2. An expanding polyvinyl alcohol sponge (Ladycon; Home Care Engros, Norway),

Reusable intravaginal ring (Introl)

A pilot laboratory study was carried out by Biswas (1988), the developer of the device, and employed a straining cystogram. Eighty-six per cent of the patients were continent with the device in place on cystogram. Following this study, the number of device sizes was increased from 8 to 25. Evaluation studies followed examining efficacy, safety and satisfaction. Davila (1996) initially demonstrated that 83% of patients were dry on pad-weight test. Later (Davila *et al.* 1999), the researchers enrolled 70 women (53 completed), aged 24–76 years, 29 with stress and 24 with mixed incontinence, in a 1-month study. A statistically significant reduction in incontinence was noted on pad testing (stress, mean 46.6 decreased to 16.6 g; mixed, mean 31.9 decreased to 6.8 g) and in bladder diary (stress, mean 28.6 decreased to 7.8 losses per week; mixed, mean 30.2 decreased to 15 losses per week); QoL scores

(I-QoL) improved in both groups. With the device in place, urodynamic testing indicated normalisation of urethral function without evidence of outflow obstruction. Subjects found the device comfortable, easy to use and convenient. Side effects include five urinary tract infections and 23 cases of vaginal soreness or mild irritation (Level of Evidence 3).

Moore *et al.* (1999a) detailed problems with both sizing and efficacy. Of the 80 recruits, 4 could not be fitted and 11 did not satisfy all entry criteria. Of the 65 participants, 39 (60%) withdrew; 20 for distorted vaginal anatomy that made fitting difficult, 5 for lack of efficacy, 4 for constipation and 10 for unrelated patient events. In the remaining 26 patients, pad-test weights decreased from a baseline median of 19 g to 2 g ($p < 0.001$), 62% were continent and 15% were $> 50\%$ improved and wished no further therapy. Moore commented that the device was difficult to fit in women who have had multiple vaginal surgeries or were oestrogen deficient. Long-term follow-up showed that 18 of 26 (from the original 65) continued to wear the device at 6 months (interim dropouts being due to concurrent illness in half and the remainder had declining efficacy). Of these, 78% continued to wear the device for a minimum follow-up of 2 years (Level of Evidence 3).

In a separate study of patients with mixed incontinence by Moore *et al.* (1999b), 5 of 21 recruits never wore the device home, leaving 16 participants. A further 2 did not reach week 4 because of poor efficacy or inability to fit the device. In the 14 who reached week 4, the median number of leaks/day declined from 4.3 to 1.0 ($p = 0.002$). Median pad-weight loss fell from 53 to 7 g ($p = 0.012$). Cystometry showed an increase in maximum bladder capacity ($p < 0.05$) and a modest reduction in severity of detrusor overactivity, with no evidence of outflow obstruction. Three women discontinued because of poor efficacy or a poorly fitting device, leaving 11 of 16 participants (69%) at week 8, when median pad weight decreased to 2 g (Level of Evidence 3).

Kondo *et al.* (1997) found no urinary flow obstruction with the device in place. Urine loss decreased from 20.6 to 4.8 g/h ($p < 0.001$) on the 60-min pad-weight test. Twenty-two patients (29%) reported complete continence, and 39 (51%) had decreased severity of incontinence by more than 50%. Minor adverse effects occurred in 26% of the patients. According to the global usefulness rating that was employed, 62 patients (81%) had some or maximum benefit (Level of Evidence 3).

Disposable intravaginal devices

Thyssen & Lose (1996) tested the Continence Guard in 26 women with stress incontinence before and after one month's use: 4 women discontinued the treatment because of discomfort or difficulties in using the device, 9 (41%) were subjectively cured of incontinence, 10 (45%) improved and 3 (14%) claimed unchanged incontinence. With the device in place, all had decreased leakage at the 24-h pad-weighing test and unchanged urodynamic tests. No vaginal or urinary infections were found (Level of Evidence 3).

Thyssen *et al.* (1999) reported on 19/22 women with stress incontinence, subjectively and objectively cured or improved in a short-term study, and who then continued the treatment with the device for 1 year. All 19 completed the study, 13 (68%) were subjectively dry, 5 (26%) were improved and 1 (5%) reported unchanged incontinence. All but one had decreased leakage on the 24-h pad test, and 67% a greater than 50% decrease. Subjective cure was 41%, and 36% were dry on the 24-h pad test. Overall reduced leakage was statistically significant ($p < 0.0005$). No significant changes were found in the other urodynamic measurements, specifically urinary flow rate.

Sander *et al.* (1999) found subjective cure in 11/55 women (20%) and improvement in 27/55 (49%) was reported. Results of the 24-h pad test and mean leakage and episodes in the voiding diary significantly decreased. After 3 months, 58% of the 55 patients desired to continue device usage. There was a highly significant improvement in QoL scores using the IIQ, as well as two additional incontinence-related QoL questionnaires. Responses to the SF-36 general health questionnaire showed no significant changes.

Hahn & Milsom (1996) reported on 121 women, in a 4-week study. Patients dropped out because of vaginal irritation (25%), other product-related reasons (6%), lack of time (6%) or failure to complete a user questionnaire. Of the remaining 90 (mean age 47.5 years), 85 performed a 24-h pad test, which showed that baseline leakage of 42 ml/24 h decreased to 14 ml/24 h ($p < 0.001$). Of these, 39 (46%) were continent. The device was considered unpleasant by 8%, and caused some local discomfort in 62% on direct questioning: 75% of these wished to continue using the device. The authors noted that older women (aged 56–65 years) tolerated the device and appeared more motivated to continue. Co-existent atrophic vaginitis and the use of topical oestrogen was not discussed

Thyssen *et al.* (2001) reported on 94 women recruited in a crossover study that compared two versions of the same device: the Conveen Continence Guard (CCG) and the Contrelle Continence Tampon (CCT). Sixty-two women (66%) completed the study with withdrawals mainly due to discomfort or for unknown reasons. Both devices reduced leakage significantly, but the CCT was significantly better than the CCG. Few side effects were reported. Thirty-two women continued the treatment for 1 year or more with 63% preferring the 'tampon'-type design for its ease of use.

The report on the polyvinyl sponge by Glavind (1997) was an acute laboratory study of only 6 women utilising a pad-test measurement during 30 min of aerobic exercise Without the vaginal sponge the patients had a mean loss of 7 g (range 2–18 g) during exercise. With the vaginal sponge *in situ* there was no leakage.

Summary

Support of the bladder neck resulting in improved continence is possible with intravaginal devices without evidence that they cause significant lower urinary tract obstruction or morbidity (Level of Evidence 3).

The reusable Introl device was shown to be an effective device for selected patients, but there were problems with sizing especially in patients with prior vaginal surgery or with vaginal atrophy. However, the device is not currently marketed.

Efficacy with the Continence Guard polyurethane expanding 'clam' device was demonstrated with selected patients and difficulties with insertion appear to have been improved by the introduction of the 'tampon'-type device. The Continence Guard device is currently marketed as Contrelle Activgard.

Studies performed in the acute setting, regardless of the device type, demonstrate better performance than diary-based studies performed over time. Efficacy is also higher in patients with minimal to moderate urinary leakage.

Relatively high dropout rates in monitored studies, during which patient support is provided, indicates the need for proper patient selection and patient and provider education (Level of Evidence 3).

- Support of the bladder neck resulting in improved continence is possible with intravaginal devices.
- Studies in acute settings demonstrate better performance than diary-based studies over time.
- Relatively high dropout rate in monitored studies.
- Long-term results not available.

Recommendations

Vaginal support devices should be included in the treatment option when managing women with SUI, dependent upon the availability of product, patient ability to manage the product (particularly manual dexterity), patient acceptance and cost (Grade of Recommendation C).

Priorities for research

Long-term results are not available and studies comparing these therapies to other forms of conservative therapy or surgery are needed.

Conclusions

Absorbent pads are the most common products used to contain urine leakage from women with unresolved incontinence. They are non-invasive, safe products which are readily available to most women. However, they contain rather than prevent urine leakage and can be bulky and obtrusive. Occlusive devices aim to prevent urine leakage and have been found to be effective in clinical trials, but are more invasive, more difficult to use and have not achieved high acceptability for patients. Only a small number of occlusive devices are actively marketed (mainly intravaginal devices) and these may be suitable for selected patients.

References

Baker, J. & Norton, P. (1996). Evaluation of absorbent products for women with mild to moderate urinary incontinence. *Applied Nursing Research* **9**, 29–33.

Balmforth, J. & Cardozo, L. D. (2003). Trends toward less invasive treatment of female stress urinary incontinence. *Urology* **62** (suppl 1), 52–60.

Bellin, P., Smith, J., Poll, W., Bogojavlensky, S., Knoll, D., Childs, S., Tuttle, J., Barada, J. & Dann, J. (1998). Results of a multicenter trial of the CapSure (Re/Stor) Continence shield on women with stress urinary incontinence. *Urology* **51**, 697–706.

Bhatia, N. N., Bergman, A. (1985). Pessary test in women with urinary incontinence. *Obstetrics and Gynecology* **65**(2), 220–6.

Biswas, N. C. (1988). A silastic vaginal device for the treatment of genuine stress incontinence. *Neurourology and Urodynamics* **7**, 271–272.

Boos, K., Anders, K., Hextall, A., Tooz-Hobson, P. & Cardozo, L. (1998). Randomised trial of Reliance versus FemAssist devices in the management of genuine stress incontinence. *Neurourology and Urodynamics*, **17**, 455–456.

Brubaker, L., Harris, T., Gleason, D., Newman, D. & North, B. (1999). The external urethral barrier for stress incontinence: a multicenter trial of safety and efficacy. Miniguard Investigators Group. *Obstetrics and Gynecology*, **93**, 932–937.

Clarke-O'Neill, S., Pettersson, L., Fader, M., Dean, G., Brooks, R. & Cottenden, A. (2002b). A multicentre comparative evaluation: washable pants with an integral pad for light incontinence. *Journal of Clinical Nursing* **11**, 79–89.

Clarke-O'Neill, S., Pettersson, L., Fader, M., Cottenden, A. & Brooks, R. (2004). A multicenter comparative evaluation: disposable pads for women with light incontinence. *Journal of Wound, Ostomy and Continence Nursing* **31**, 32–42.

Davila, G. W. (1996). Introl bladder neck support prosthesis: a nonsurgical urethropexy. *Journal of Endourology* **10**, 293–296.

Davila, G. W., Neal, D., Horbach, N., Peacher, J., Doughtie, J. D., Karram, M. (1999). A bladder-neck support prosthesis for women with stress and mixed incontinence. *Obstetrics and Gynecology* **93**(6) 938–42.

Dunn, M., Brandt, D. & Nygaard, I. (2002). Treatment of exercise incontinence with a urethral insert: a pilot study. *The Physician and Sports Medicine* **30**, 45–51.

Eckford, S. D., Jackson, S. R., Lewis, P. A. & Abrams, P. (1996). The continence control pad: a new external urethral occlusion device in the management of stress incontinence. *British Journal of Urology* **77**, 538–540.

Glavind, K. (1997). Use of a vaginal sponge during aerobic exercises in patients with stress urinary incontinence. *International Urogynecology Journal and Pelvic Floor Dysfunction* **8**, 351–353.

Hahn, I. & Milsom, I. (1996). Treatment of female stress urinary incontinence with a new anatomically shaped vaginal device (Conveen Continence Guard). *British Journal of Urology* **77**, 711–715.

Kondo, A., Yokoyama, E., Koshiba, K., Fukui, J., Gotoh, M., Yoshikawa, Y., Yamada, T. & Takei, M. (1997). Bladder neck support prosthesis: a nonoperative treatment for stress or mixed urinary incontinence. *Journal of Urology* **157**, 824–827.

Miller, J. L. & Bavendam, T. (1996). Treatment with the Reliance urinary control insert: one-year experience. *Journal of Endourology* **10**, 287–292.

Moore, K. H., Foote, A., Burton, G. & King, J. (1999a). An open study of the bladder neck support prosthesis in genuine stress incontinence. *British Journal of Obstetrics and Gynaecology* **106**, 42–49.

Moore, K. H., Simons, A., Dowell, C., Bryant, C. & Prashar, S. (1999b). Efficacy and user acceptability of the urethral occlusive device in women with urinary incontinence. *Journal of Urology* **162**, 464–468.

Nielsen, K. K., Walter, S., Maegaard, E. & Kromann-Andersen, B. (1993). The urethral plug II: an alternative treatment in women with genuine urinary stress incontinence. *British Journal of Urology* **72**, 428–432.

Nygaard, I. (1995). Prevention of exercise incontinence with mechanical devices. *Journal of Reproductive Medicine* **40**, 89–94.

Peschers, U., Zen, R. F., Schaer, G. N. & Schussler, B. (1996). The VIVA urethral plug: a sensible expansion of the spectrum for conservative therapy of urinary stress incontinence? *Geburtshilfe Frauenheilkd.* **56**, 118–123.

Realini, J. P. & Walters, M. D. (1990). Vaginal diaphragm rings in the treatment of stress urinary incontinence. *Journal of the American Board of Family Practice* **3**, 99–103.

Sand, P. K., Staskin, D., Miller, J., Diokno, A., Sant, G. R., Davila, G. W., Knapp, P., Rappaport, S. & Tutrone, R. (1999). Effect of a urinary control insert on quality of life in incontinent women. *International Urogynecology Journal and Pelvic Floor Dysfunction* **10**, 100–105.

Sander, P., Thyssen, H., Lose, G. & Andersen, J. T. (1999). Effect of a vaginal device on quality of life with urinary stress incontinence. *Obstetrics and Gynecology* **93**, 407–411.

Shinopulos, N. M., Dann, J. A. & Smith, J. J. III (1999). Patient selection and education for use of the CapSure (Re/Stor) continence shield. *Urologic Nursing* **19**, 135–140.

Staskin, D., Bavendam, T., Miller, J., Davila, G. W., Diokno, A., Knapp, P., Rappaport, S., Sand, P., Sant, G. & Tutrone, R. (1996). Effectiveness of a urinary control insert in the management of stress urinary incontinence: early results of a multicenter study. *Urology* **47**, 629–636.

Suarez, G. M., Baum, N. H. & Jacobs, J. (1991). Use of standard contraceptive diaphragm in management of stress urinary incontinence. *Urology* **37**, 119–122.

Thornburn, P., Fader, M., Dean, G., Brooks, R. & Cottenden, A. (1997). Improving the performance of small incontinence pads: a study of 'wet comfort'. *Journal of Wound, Ostomy and Continence Nursing* **24**, 219–225.

Thyssen, H. & Lose, G. (1996). New disposable vaginal device (continence guard) in the treatment of female stress incontinence. Design, efficacy and short term safety. *Acta Obstetricia et Gynecologica Scandinavica* **75**, 170–173.

Thyssen, H., Sander, P. & Lose, G. (1999). A vaginal device (continence guard) in the management of urge incontinence in women. *International Urogynecology Journal and Pelvic Floor Dysfunction* **10**, 219–222.

Thyssen, H., Bidmead, J., Lose, G., Moller, B. K., Dwyer, P. & Cardozo, L. (2001). A new intravaginal device for stress incontinence in women. *BJU International* **88**, 889–892.

Tincello, D. G., Adams, E. J., Bolderson, J., Richmond, D. H. (2000). A urinary control device for management of female stress incontinence. *Obstetrics and Gynecology* **95 (3)**, 417–20.

Tincello, D. G., Bolderson, J. & Richmond, D. H. (1997). Preliminary experience with a urinary control device in the management of women with genuine stress incontinence, *British Journal of Urology* **80**, 752–756.

Versi, E. & Harvey, M. A. (1998). Efficacy of an external urethral device in women with genuine stress urinary incontinence. *International Urogynecology Journal and Pelvic Floor Dysfunction* **9**, 271–274.

Chapter 10

The evidence base for medical intervention in stress urinary incontinence

Matthew Parsons, Dudley Robinson and Linda Cardozo

Introduction

Urodynamic stress incontinence is the commonest cause of urinary incontinence in women in the United Kingdom, and represents around 50% of diagnoses. An epidemiological survey of 29,500 households across four European countries also showed that stress urinary incontinence is the commonest presenting symptom with 42% of respondents admitting to stress-type leakage in the preceding 30 days (Hanskaar *et al.* 2004).

Clinical features

Stress urinary incontinence (SUI) is the involuntary leakage of urine from the urethra, synchronous with effort or exertion, or sneezing or coughing (Abrams *et al.* 2002). The urine is usually lost in small amounts, without any associated urgency. 25% of incontinent women suffer incontinence during sexual intercourse. This usually occurs at penetration, rather than orgasm, in women complaining of SUI (Hilton 1998).

Overall, approximately half of all incontinent women complain of pure stress incontinence and 30–40% of mixed symptoms of stress and urge incontinence (Hannestad *et al.* 2000).

Definition

Urodynamic stress incontinence (as opposed to the patient symptom 'stress incontinence') is only diagnosed after performing urodynamics, and is the involuntary leakage of urine per urethram during episodes of raised intra-abdominal pressure, in the absence of a detrusor contraction (Abrams *et al.* 2002).

Treatment of urodynamic stress incontinence

Conservative Management

A conservative approach is often justified, especially if symptoms are only mild, or easily manageable. When a woman's family is incomplete, or when symptoms manifest during pregnancy or immediately afterwards, surgery should be avoided. If surgery is considered unwise because of medical illness, when surgery is refused, or if the waiting time for surgery is long, the symptoms may be ameliorated by appropriate, conservative interventions.

Physiotherapy

The mainstay of treatment for USI, in the United Kingdom, has always been physiotherapy, with recourse to surgery when indicated and desired. Physiotherapy represents the least invasive, effective option for treating stress urinary incontinence. Pelvic floor exercise (PFE) is more effective than no treatment, electrical stimulation, and vaginal cones (Bo et al. 1999). The advantage of this approach is that many women's symptoms are cured or improved to the point where they do not require surgery, with its potential complications (Jarvis 1994). Additionally, the success rate of future operative procedures is not adversely affected by pelvic floor exercises, as it may be following failed surgical treatment.

Some women express a preference for surgery as they are attracted by the more 'rapid' success rate (Karantanis et al. 2003). As a first procedure, sub-urethral slings and colposuspension can both be expected to have a success rate of around 90% (Jarvis 1994), although they are also associated with both peri-operative and postoperative complications. A pharmacological agent, either alone, or in combination with physical therapy, may represent an attractive alternative to physiotherapy or surgery.

Drug Therapy

Until very recently, there were no pharmacological agents available for the management of urodynamic stress incontinence, although various drugs such as α_1–adrenoceptor agonists, oestrogens, and tricyclic antidepressants have all been used anecdotally in the past. Consequently, there remains a need for a safe, effective drug for the management of urodynamic stress incontinence.

In this chapter, we discuss the evidence pertaining to the use of phenyl-propanolamine (an $\alpha 1$–adrenoceptor agonist), imipramine (a tricyclic antidepressant), oestrogens, desmopressin, and duloxetine (a new, balanced, serotonin and noradrenaline re-uptake inhibitor).

α1-adrenoceptor agonists

The storage reflex

During the micturition cycle, the nervous mechanisms for co-ordinating storage and emptying of urine involve sympathetic, parasympathetic, and somatic nerves, in a complex series of reflex pathways. There is normally a reciprocal arrangement of contraction and relaxation between the bladder and outlet structures, such that during filling, bladder relaxation is accompanied by urethral sphincter contraction; during voiding, bladder contraction occurs simultaneously with sphincter relaxation to facilitate bladder emptying (Andersson et al. 2001).

During filling, the bladder has to relax to allow low pressure filling. Stretch receptors pass information about bladder filling via the somatic nerves travelling in the pelvic nerve (Elbadawi 1986). There is little evidence in humans of a direct sympathetic innervation to the detrusor muscle. Rather, sympathetic fibres travelling via the hypogastric nerve are stimulated in the upper lumbar region, and provide α_1-adrenergic stimulation to the urethral sphincter, maintaining its closure in the filling phase (deGroat 1999). α1-adrenoceptor agonists have thus been used to try and improve urethral sphincter contraction in patients with urinary incontinence.

Phenylpropanolamine

Three studies have compared the effect of phenylpropanolamine (PPA), an α_1-adrenoceptor agonist, with placebo in the management of urodynamic stress incontinence (Collste & Lindskog 1987; Fossberg et al. 1983; Lehtonen et al. 1986). One other study (Kinn & Lindskog 1988) treated all participants with PPA before comparing the effect of placebo or oestriol given additionally.

Lehtonen et al. (1986) undertook a randomised, double-blind, placebo controlled trial of PPA 50 mg BD, in 43 women with mild to moderate USI over a two week study period. Subjective outcome was significantly better on PPA (15 of 21 reporting improvement, compared with 8 of 22 in the placebo arm, $p = 0.01$). Significant increase in the maximum urethral closure pressure (MUCP) of 14% was seen in the PPA group, but no significant correlation was seen with subjective outcome. Both arms were found to have a increase in functional urethral length, but no significant difference between them. Significant adverse reactions were noted to be rare.

Fossberg et al. (1983) studied the effect of PPA 50 mg BD and placebo, in 23 females with USI. Three patients dropped out, of whom one dropped out because of side effects. Twelve patients reported subjective improvement on PPA, and three on placebo. None became continent. Objective assessment demonstrated a rise in MUCP on PPA, but this was not related to serum concentration.

Collste and Lindskog (1987) performed a randomised, double-blind, placebo-controlled, cross-over study of the effect of two weeks treatment of PPA 50 mg BD in 24 women with mild to moderate USI. PPA caused a significant increase in MUCP, but no change in functional urethral length. In our unit, we often find that women with USI report urgency and habitual frequency, purportedly because of urine in the proximal urethra (Balmforth et al. 2003). Treatment with PPA might therefore reduce such urgency/frequency symptoms. However, although leakage episodes were significantly reduced, urinary frequency remained unchanged (Collste & Lindskog 1987). Adverse reactions were few and negligible.

The use of PPA in combination with oestrogens is discussed later in this chapter. However, Kinn & Lindskog (1988) recruited 36 post-menopausal women with USI to their study comparing PPA with PPA and oestriol in combination. All, however, received a four-week, single-blind regime of PPA 50 mg BD.

Significant reduction in the leakage amount was seen after treatment with PPA ($p = 0.05$).

Twenty-two of the thirty women who completed the study reported side effects of dry mouth, insomnia, tiredness, irritability, depression, flush, constipation, nausea, and/or arthralgia, in 36 of the 90 treatment periods. A probable relation to PPA could be established only in two cases with dryness of mouth and in one case with constipation, as they were reported in both treatment periods including PPA. This low frequency could not be separated from placebo effects and long-term maintenance medication. PPA has been withdrawn from the market in the USA owing to a risk of stroke.

Imipramine

Imipramine is a tricyclic anti-depressant that has been used in the treatment of incontinence in two different ways. Because of its marked antimuscarinic side effects, it has been used in the treatment of detrusor overactivity, and has been especially used where nocturia is a problem. It has also been used in the treatment of stress incontinence, because it functions as a serotonin and noradrenaline re-uptake inhibitor, and so should increase the tone of urethral smooth muscle (Andersson et al. 2002). In theory, it should also increase the tone in the striated muscle of the urethra and pelvic floor by augmentation at Onuf's nucleus. It is the latter use that we shall consider in this chapter.

Gilja et al. (1984) administered 75 mg imipramine daily to 30 women with USI, for four weeks. A total of 21 women (71%) stated that they were continent after treatment with imipramine, and had an increased mean MUCP from 34 to 48 mm Hg, while 9 (29%) did not improve and treatment was stopped. Imipramine extended the functional urethral length and made it independent of stress factors in women who were continent after treatment with imipramine. In patients with persistent incontinence the functional urethral length was extended significantly, but was shortened with stress despite imipramine therapy.

Lin et al. (1999) have reported the use of imipramine in an open study involving 40 women with USI. Each received 75 mg imipramine daily for three months. After treatment, 35% ($n = 14$) were cured, 25% ($n = 10$) improved by at least 50% and in the remaining 40% ($n = 16$) treatment failed. The efficacy of successful treatment was 60% (95% confidence interval (CI) 44.8–75.2).

Outcome did not seem to be dependent on age, parity, or hormonal status and the only urodynamic variables to differ between treatment success and failure groups were MUCP (77 cm H_2O (intraquantile range (IQR) 61–105) for the treatment success group versus 40 cm H_2O (IQR 34–53) in the treatment failure group ($p < 0.0001$) and functional urethral length (median functional urethral length was 3 cm (IQR 2.3–3) in the treatment success group versus 2.3 cm (IQR 2–3) in the treatment failure group ($p = 0.028$)).

No placebo-controlled, randomised trials involving imipramine have been reported and so its use cannot be advocated. Additionally, it has been associated with falls in the elderly and so should certainly be avoided in that population.

Oestrogens

Oestrogens and lower urinary tract function

Oestrogens may play an important role in the continence mechanism with bladder and urethral function becoming less efficient with age (Rud *et al.* 1980). Elderly women have been found to have a reduced flow rate, increased urinary residuals, higher filling pressures, reduced bladder capacity and lower maximum voiding pressures (Malone-Lee 1988). Oestrogens may affect continence by increasing urethral resistance, raising the sensory threshold of the bladder (Fantl *et al.* 1988) or by increasing α-adrenoceptor sensitivity in the urethral smooth muscle and thereby increasing tone (Kinn & Lindskog 1988; Versi & Cardozo 1988). In addition, exogenous oestrogens have been shown to increase the number of intermediate and superficial cells in the vagina of postmenopausal women (Smith 1976) and these changes have also been demonstrated in the bladder and urethra (Samsioe *et al.* 1985).

Bladder function

Oestrogen receptors, although absent in the transitional epithelium of the bladder are present in the areas of the trigone which have undergone squamous metaplasia (Kinn & Lindskog 1988). Oestrogen is known to have a direct effect on detrusor function— oestradiol has been shown to reduce the amplitude and frequency of spontaneous rhythmic detrusor contractions (Shenfield *et al.* 1998).

Urethra

Oestrogen receptors have been demonstrated in the squamous epithelium of both the proximal and distal urethra (Kinn & Lindskog 1988) and oestrogen has been shown to improve the maturation index of urethral squamous epithelium (Bergman *et al.* 1990). It has been suggested that oestrogen increases urethral closure pressure and improves pressure transmission to the proximal urethra, both promoting continence (Bhatia *et al.* 1989; Hilton & Stanton 1983; Karram *et al.* 1989; Rud 1980)

Lower urinary tract symptoms

Epidemiological studies have implicated oestrogen deficiency in the aetiology of lower urinary tract symptoms with 70% of women relating the onset of urinary incontinence to their final menstrual period (Iosif & Bekassy 1984). Lower urinary tract symptoms are common in postmenopausal women attending a menopause clinic with 20% complaining of severe urgency and almost 50% complaining of stress incontinence (Cardozo *et al.* 1987). Urge incontinence in particular is more prevalent following the menopause and the prevalence would appear to rise with increasing years of oestrogen deficiency (Kondo et al. 1990). There is, however, conflicting evidence regarding the role of oestrogen withdrawal at the time of the menopause. Some studies have shown a peak incidence in perimenopausal women (Jolleys 1988; Thomas et al. 1980), while other evidence suggests that many women develop incontinence at least 10 years before the cessation of menstruation with significantly more premenopausal women than postmenopausal women being affected (Burgio et al. 1991; Samicoe 1998).

Urinary tract infection is also a common cause of urinary symptoms in women of all ages. This is a particular problem in the elderly with a reported incidence of 20% in the community and over 50% in institutionalised patients (Boscia & Kaye 1987; Sandford 1975). Pathophysiological changes such as impairment of bladder emptying, poor perineal hygiene and both faecal and urinary incontinence may partly account for the high prevalence observed. In addition, as previously described, changes in the vaginal flora due to oestrogen depletion lead to colonisation with gram negative bacilli, which in addition to causing local irritative symptoms also act as uropathogens. These microbiological changes may be reversed with oestrogen replacement following the menopause, which offer a rationale for treatment and prophylaxis.

Urogenital atrophy

Withdrawal of endogenous oestrogen at the menopause results in well-documented climacteric symptoms such as hot flushes and night sweats in addition to the less commonly reported symptoms of urogenital atrophy. Symptoms do not usually develop until several years following the menopause when levels of endogenous oestrogens fall below the level required to promote endometrial growth (Samicoe 1998). This temporal relationship would suggest oestrogen withdrawal as the cause.

The Hormones and Urogenital Therapy (HUT) Committee have performed a review of oestrogen therapy in the management of urogenital atrophy (Cardozo et al. 1998). Meta-analysis of ten placebo-controlled trials confirmed the significant effect of oestrogens in the management of urogenital atrophy. Oestrogen is efficacious in the treatment of urogenital atrophy and low dose vaginal preparations are as effective as systemic therapy.

Oestrogens in the management of incontinence

Oestrogen preparations have been used for many years in the treatment of urinary incontinence (Salmon et al. 1941; Youngblood et al. 1957), although their precise role remains controversial. Many of the studies performed have been uncontrolled observational series examining the use of a wide range of different preparations, doses and routes of administration. The inconsistent use of progestogens to provide endometrial protection is a further confounding factor making interpretation of the results difficult.

To clarify the situation a meta-analysis from the HUT Committee has been reported (Fantl *et al.* 1994). Of 166 articles identified, which were published in English between 1969 and 1992, only six were controlled trials and 17 were uncontrolled series. Meta-analysis found an overall significant effect of oestrogen therapy on subjective improvement in all subjects and for subjects with urodynamic stress incontinence alone. However, when assessing objective fluid loss there was no significant effect. Maximum urethral closure pressure was found to increase significantly with oestrogen therapy although this outcome was influenced by a single study showing a large effect (Henalla *et al.* 1989).

A Cochrane review of the use of oestrogens to treat urinary incontinence considered 15 trials that compared oestrogen with placebo during which 374 women received oestrogen and 344 placebo (Moehrer *et al.* 2003). When subjective cure and improvement are considered together, a statistically higher cure and improvement rate was shown for stress incontinence (46/107, 43% versus 29/109, 27%). For women with urge incontinence, the chance of cure or improvement was approximately a quarter higher again than in women with stress incontinence. Combined oestrogen and progesterone appeared to reduce the likelihood of cure or improvement.

Oestrogens in the management of stress incontinence

In addition to the studies included in the HUT meta-analysis, several authors have also investigated the role of oestrogen therapy in the management of urodynamic stress incontinence only. Oral oestrogens have been reported to increase the maximum urethral pressures and lead to symptomatic improvement in 65–70% of women (Caine & Raz 1973; Rud 1980), although other work has not confirmed this (Walter *et al.* 1978; Wilson *et al.* 1987).

A recently reported meta-analysis has helped determine the role of oestrogen replacement in women with stress incontinence (Ahmed Al-Badr *et al.* 2003). Interestingly, there was only a symptomatic or clinical improvement noted in the non-randomised studies whereas there was no such effect noted in the randomised trials.

From the available evidence oestrogen does not appear to be an effective treatment for stress incontinence although it may have a synergistic role in combination therapy.

Two placebo-controlled studies have examined the use of oral and vaginal oestrogens with the a-adrenergic agonist, phenylpropanolamine (PPA), used separately and in combination. Both studies found that combination therapy was superior to either drug given alone, although whereas there was subjective improvement in all groups (Beisland *et al.* 1984) there was only objective improvement in the combination therapy group (Hilton *et al.* 1990). Two further studies compared oestrogen alone or oestrogen and PPA in combination (Alstrom *et al.* 1990; Kinn & Lindskog 1988), and demonstrated an additional effect of PPA in reducing the urinary leakage episode frequency, in comparison with oestrogen alone.

Such combination therapy may offer an alternative conservative treatment for women who have mild urodynamic stress incontinence although there are safety concerns regarding PPA and it has been withdrawn in USA.

Selective oestrogen receptor modulators (SERMS)

A recent development in hormonal therapy has been the development of selective oestrogen receptor modulators (SERMS). These drugs have oestrogen like actions in maintaining bone density and in lowering serum cholesterol but have anti-oestrogenic effects on the breast (Park & Jordan 2002) and do not cause endometrial stimulation (Silfen *et al.* 1999). Early work suggests that some SERMS in development, levormeloxifene and idoxifene, might increase the risk of urogenital prolapse (Hendrix & McNeeley 2001), although there were some methodological problems noted in the study. However, in an analysis of three randomised, double-blind, placebo controlled trials investigating raloxifene in 6926 postmenopausal women, there appeared to be a protective effect, with fewer treated women having surgery for urogenital prolapse; 1.5% versus 0.75% ($p < 0.005$) (Goldstein *et al.* 2001). At present, the long-term effect of SERMS on the urogenital tract remains to be determined and there are few data regarding effects on urinary incontinence.

Desmopressin

Anti-diuretic hormone (ADH) allows increased tubular reabsorption of urine and so reduces urine output from the kidney. Production shows a diurnal variation and loss of production, more common in the elderly, is associated with nocturnal polyuria.

Desmopressin, a nonapeptide analogue of ADH, is available as a nasal insufflation or tablet form, and is licensed for the treatment of paediatric and adult nocturnal enuresis. As an unlicensed use, it may be useful in the management of stress urinary incontinence to reduce urine production selectively at certain times of the day, allowing women to continue with their normal activities.

A multicentre, multinational, randomised, double-blind, placebo-controlled, cross-over exploratory study of 60 women, aged 18–80 years, complaining of severe daytime urinary incontinence was conducted (Robinson *et al.* 2004), of whom 57 completed the study. There was a higher incidence of periods with no leakage in the first four hours and during the first eight hours on desmopressin than on placebo. There was also a higher frequency of dry days on desmopressin than on placebo; 36% of patients had no leakage on virtually all treatment days (6 or 7) for four hours after dosing. There were no serious or severe adverse events reported. Seven women (11%) withdrew from the study, of whom five did not attend for the final visit and two (3%) because of mild adverse events.

The results of the study suggest that the use of desmopressin is safe and effective in the management of daytime incontinence, when used as a 'designer' drug specifically to target therapy to cover important daytime events.

Editors' note: the reader is referred to p.139 for additional data on oestrogen replacement therapy which we included immediately before going to press.

Duloxetine

A new drug has been marketed, specifically for the treatment of stress incontinence. Duloxetine is a potent and balanced serotonin (5-hydroxytryptamine) and noradrenaline reuptake inhibitor (SNRI) that enhances urethral striated sphincter activity via a centrally mediated pathway (Thor & Katofiasc 1995).

The efficacy and safety of duloxetine (20 mg, 40 mg, 80 mg) has been evaluated in a double-blind randomised parallel group placebo controlled phase II dose finding study in 48 centres in the USA involving 553 women with stress incontinence (Norton *et al*. 2002). Duloxetine was associated with significant and dose dependent decreases in incontinence episode frequency. Reductions were 41% for placebo and 54%, 59% and 64% for the 20 mg, 40 mg and 80 mg groups respectively. Discontinuation rates were also dose dependent; 5% for placebo and 9%, 12% and 15% of 20 mg, 40 mg and 80 mg respectively, the most frequently reported adverse event being nausea.

A further global phase III randomised study of 458 women has also recently been reported (Millard *et al*. 2003). There was a significant decrease in incontinence episode frequency and improvement in quality of life in those women taking duloxetine 40 mg BD when compared to placebo. Once again, nausea was the most frequently reported adverse event occurring in 25.1% of women receiving duloxetine compared to a rate of 3.9% in those taking placebo. However, 60% of nausea resolved by 7 days and 86% by one month.

These findings are supported by a further double blind, placebo controlled study of 109 women awaiting surgery for stress incontinence (Drutz *et al*. 2003). Overall, there was a significant improvement in incontinence episode frequency and quality of life in those women taking duloxetine when compared to placebo. Furthermore, 33.3% admitted to being much better, or very much better, and 20% of women who were awaiting continence surgery changed their mind whilst taking duloxetine.

Van Kerrebroeck *et al*. (2004) conducted a randomised, double-blind, placebo-controlled trial comparing duloxetine 80 mg/day and placebo, in European and Canadian women. The study included 494 women aged 24–83 years of age, with predominant symptoms of stress urinary incontinence, using a clinical algorithm that was highly predictive of USI in a small subgroup of 34 women.

Incontinence episode frequency was significantly reduced in comparison with the placebo arm [median decrease 50% versus 29%, $p = 0.002$]. There was also comparable improvement in the women most severely affected, with more than 14 incontinence episodes per week [median decrease 56% versus 27%, $p < 0.001$].

Discontinuation was higher in the duloxetine arm of the study (22% versus 5%, $p < 0.001$) with the commonest reason for discontinuation being nausea (5.3%).

These findings were mirrored in a study of 683 North American women (Dmochowski *et al*. 2003) with predominant stress urinary incontinence, positive cough stress test and pad test and a bladder capacity greater than 400 mls. There was a significant decrease in incontinence episode frequency with duloxetine (50% versus

27%, $p < 0.001$) with comparable improvements in quality of life, as assessed by I-QoL (11 versus 6.8, $p < 0.001$). 51% of duloxetine patients were >50% IEF-responders, compared with 34% of placebo patients; concomitant increase in voiding interval on duloxetine was noted (20 minutes versus 2 minutes, $p < 0.001$).

Discontinuation rates were 24% for duloxetine and 4% for placebo ($p < 0.001$) with nausea being the commonest reason (6.4%). Of the 78 women who experienced treatment-emergent nausea, 58 (74%) completed the study.

Duloxetine has been cited by many clinicians as being a useful adjunct to physiotherapy. In one 12-week study in 201 women, women were randomised to duloxetine plus pelvic floor muscle exercises, pelvic floor muscles exercises alone or placebo. Duloxetine, with or without PFMT, was superior to PFMT alone or placebo. Quality of life analyses suggested greater improvement with combined treatment (Ghomeni, 2005). The safety of duloxetine has been evaluated and summarised after four 12-week placebo-controlled clinical trials, and includes 958 duloxetine-treated patients, and 955 placebo-treated patients (Duloxetine, summary of product characteristics). This represents 190 patient years of exposure to duloxetine at 40 mg BD. The commonest adverse effects were nausea, dry mouth, fatigue, insomnia, and constipation (see Table 10.1).

Table 10.1 Summary of common side effects (at least 10% of users)

System Organ Class	Adverse Event	Duloxetine n = 958 (%)	Placebo n = 955 (%)
Psychiatric disorders	Insomnia	12.6	1.9
Gastro-intestinal disorders	Nausea	23.2	3.7
	Dry mouth	13.4	1.5
	Constipation	11.0	2.3
General disorders and administration site conditions	Fatigue	12.7	3.8

Conclusions

PPA is given to provide positive reinforcement of α-adrenergic stimulation of the urethral sphincter that is normal in the filling phase of the micturition cycle.

PPA has been shown to subjectively improve symptoms and is well tolerated in all of the small studies in which it has been used. Although there have been some objective changes in urodynamic variables, namely urethral closure pressure, there is no evidence that MUCP is significantly correlated with subjective improvement. No patients in the studies were continent and dry after treatment with PPA. It has also been associated with an increased risk of stroke. For these reasons it has fallen out of favour in recent years.

Only two small open studies of the use of imipramine have been undertaken, involving very small numbers of women. The efficacy was found to be of the order of 60%. On the basis of current evidence, its use cannot be advocated outside of clinical trials, especially in the light of problems with falls in the elderly.

Oestrogens are known to have an important physiological effect on the female lower genital tract throughout adult life leading to symptomatic, histological and functional changes. Urogenital atrophy is the manifestation of oestrogen withdrawal following the menopause, presenting with vaginal and/or urinary symptoms. The use of oestrogen replacement therapy has been examined in the management of lower urinary tract symptoms as well as in the treatment of urogenital atrophy, although only recently has it been subjected to randomised placebo controlled trials and meta-analysis.

Oestrogen therapy alone has been shown to have little effect in the management of urodynamic stress incontinence. It has, however, been shown to improve outcome of treatment with PPA, and future studies of duloxetine may study the effect of combination treatment in the same manner.

Desmopressin represents a safe and effective treatment modality for the management of daytime urinary incontinence, by reducing urine output. Users are more likely to have no incontinence episodes in the first four hours after use, and more likely to have a 'dry day' after use.

Duloxetine represents the first pharmacological agent developed specifically for the treatment of stress urinary incontinence. It has been shown to be effective even with moderate and severe symptoms. The commonest side effect is nausea, but this is usually mild to moderate, and transient. Discontinuation rates are very low, with nausea symptoms improving within a month or so.

The onset of action is rapid with duloxetine – studies have demonstrated efficacy within a few weeks – and appears to be sustained. It may be that duloxetine used in combination with physiotherapy offers an excellent combination of more rapid improvement, sustained over time by improved pelvic floor muscle strength after physiotherapy.

The mainstay of treatment for stress urinary incontinence remains physical therapy. However, for those women who fail to respond satisfactorily, duloxetine may offer an effective alternative to surgery and pelvic floor education in the management of women with moderate to severe stress incontinence.

References

Abrams, P., Cardozo, L., Fall, M. *et al.* (2002). The Standardisation of Terminology of Lower Urinary Tract Function: Report from the Standardisation Sub-Committee of the International Continence Society. *Neurourology and Urodynamics* **21**, 167–178.

Ahlstrom, K., Sandahl, B., Sjoberg, B., Ulmsten, U., Stormby, N. & Lindskog, M. (1990). Effect of combined treatment with phenylpropanolamine and estriol, compared with estriol treatment alone, in postmenopausal women with stress urinary incontinence. *Gynecologic and Obstetric Investigation* **30**, 37–43.

Ahmed, Al-Badr, Ross, S., Soroka, D. & Drutz, H. P. (2003). What is the available evidence for hormone replacement therapy in women with stress urinary incontinence? *Journal of Obstetrics and Gynaecology Canada* **25**, 567–574.

Andersson, K. E. & Waldeck, K. (2001). Pharmacology of the bladder. In *Textbook of Female Urology and Urogynaecology* (ed. L. Cardozo & D. Staskin, D.), pp. 139–150. Oxford: Isis Medical Media.

Andersson, K.-E. *et al.* (2002). Pharmacological treatment of urinary incontinence. In *Incontinence. 2nd International Consultation on Incontinence, July 1–3, 2001*, second edition (ed. P. Abrams, L. D. Cardozo, S. Khoury & A. Wein), pp. 479–511. Plymouth, UK. Health Publication Ltd.

Balmforth, J., Bidmead, J. & Cardozo, L. (2003). The effect of fluid entering the proximal urethra on detrusor pressure and the subjective sensation of urge. In *Proceedings of the 33rd Annual Meeting of the International Continence Society. Florence, Italy. October 2003.* Abstract 163.

Beisland, H. O., Fossberg, E., Moer, A. *et al.* (1984). Urethral insufficiency in post-menopausal females: treatment with phenylpropanolamine and oestriol separately and in combination. *Urologia Internationalis* **39**, 211–216.

Bergman, A., Karram, M. M. & Bhatia, N. N. (1990). Changes in urethral cytology following oestrogen administration. *Gynecologic and Obstetric Investigation* **29**, 211–213.

Bhatia, N. N., Bergman, A., Karram, M. M. *et al.* (1989). Effects of oestrogen on urethral function in women with urinary incontinence. *American Journal of Obstetrics and Gynecology* **160**, 176–180

Bo, K., Talseth, T. & Holme, I. (1999). Single blind, randomised controlled trial of pelvic floor exercises, electrical stimulation, vaginal cones, and no treatment in management of genuine stress incontinence in women. *British Medical Journal* **318**, 487–493.

Boscia, J. A. & Kaye, D. (1987). Asymptomatic bacteria in the elderly. *Infectious Disease Clinics of North America* **1**, 893–903.

Burgio, K. L., Matthews, K. A. & Engel, B. (1991). Prevalence, incidence and correlates of urinary incontinence in healthy, middle aged women. *Journal of Urology* **146**, 1255–1259.

Caine, M. & Raz, S. (1973) The role of female hormones in stress incontinence. In *Proceedings of the 19th Congress of the International Society of Urology, Amsterdam, The Netherlands.*

Cardozo, L.D., Bachmann, G., McClish, D., Fonda, D. & Birgerson, L. (1998). Meta-analysis of oestrogen therapy in the management of urogenital atrophy in postmenopausal women: Second report of the Hormones and Urogenital Therapy Committee. *Obstetrics and Gynecology* **92**, 722–727.

Cardozo, L. D., Tapp, A., Versi, E., Samsioe, G. & Bonne Erickson, P. (eds) (1987). The lower urinary tract in peri- and postmenopausal women. In *The Urogenital Deficiency Syndrome*, pp. 10–17. Bagsverd, Denmark: Novo Industri AS.

Collste, L. & Lindskog, M. (1987). Phenylpropanolamine in treatment of female stress urinary incontinence. Double-blind placebo controlled study in 24 patients. *Urology* **30**, 398–403.

deGroat, W. C. (1999). Basic neurophysiology and neuropharmacology. In *Incontinence* (ed. P. Abrams *et al.*), pp. 105–154. Plymouth, UK. Health Publication Ltd.

Dmochowski, R. R., Miklos, J. R., Norton, P. A., Zumner, N. R., Yalcin, I., Bump, R. C. *et al.* (2003). Duloxetine versus placebo for the treatment of North American women with stress urinary incontinence. *Journal of Urology* **170**, 1259–1263.

Drutz, H., Cardozo, L., Baygani, S. & Bump, R. (2003). Duloxetine treatment of women with only urodynamic stress incontinence awaiting continence surgery. *Neurourology and Urodynamics* **22**, 523–524.

Elbadawi, A. (1986). Neuromuscular mechanisms of micturition. In *Neurourology and Urodynamics: Principles & Practice*, (ed. S. V. Yalla *et al.*), New York: Macmillan.

Fantl, J. A., Wyman, J. F., Anderson, R. L. *et al.* (1988). Postmenopausal urinary incontinence: comparison between non-oestrogen and oestrogen supplemented women. *Obstetrics and Gynecology* **71**, 823–828.

Fantl, J. A., Cardozo, L. D., McClish, D. K. and the Hormones and Urogenital Therapy Committee. (1994). Oestrogen therapy in the management of incontinence in postmenopausal women: a meta-analysis. First report of the Hormones and Urogenital Therapy Committee. *Obstetrics and Gynecology* **83**, 12–18.

Fossberg, E., Beisland, H. O. & Lundgren, R. A. (1983). Stress incontinence in females: treatment with phenylpropanolamine. A urodynamic and pharmacological evaluation. *Urologia Internationalis* **38**, 293–299.

Ghomeni, G. L. *et al.* (2005). *Journal of Urology* **173 (5)** 1647–1653.

Gilja, I., Radej, M., Kovacic, M. & Parazajder, J. (1984). Conservative treatment of female stress incontinence with imipramine *Journal of Urology* **132**, 909–911.

Goldstein, S. R., Neven, P., Zhou, L., Taylor, Y. L., Ciacca, A. V. & Plouffe, L. (2001). Raloxifene effect on frequency of surgery for pelvic floor relaxation. *Obstetrics and Gynecology* **98**, 91–96.

Hannestad, Y. S., Rortveit, G., Sandvik, H. & Hunskaar, S. (2000). A community-based epidemiological survey of female urinary incontinence: the Norwegian EPINCONT study. Epidemiology of incontinence in the county of Nord-Trondelag. *Journal of Clinical Epidemiology* **53**, 1150–1157.

Henalla, S. M., Hutchins, C. J., Robinson, P. & Macivar, J. (1989). Non –operative methods in the treatment of female genuine stress incontinence of urine. *British Journal of Obstetrics and Gynaecology* **9**, 222–225.

Hendrix, S. L. & McNeeley, S. G. (2001). Effect of selective oestrogen receptor modulators on reproductive tissues other than endometrium. *Annals of the New York Academy of Sciences* **949**, 243–250.

Hilton, P. (1988) Urinary incontinence during sexual intercourse: a common, but rarely volunteered, symptom. *British Journal of Obstetrics and Gynaecology* **95**, 377–381.

Hilton, P. & Stanton, S. L. (1983). The use of intravaginal oestrogen cream in genuine stress incontinence. *British Journal of Obstetrics and Gynaecology* **90**, 940–944.

Hilton, P., Tweddel, A. L. & Mayne, C. (1990). Oral and intravaginal oestrogens alone and in combination with alpha-adrenergic stimulation in genuine stress incontinence. *International Urogynecology Journal* **12**, 80–86.

Hunskaar, S., Lose, G., Sykes, D. & Voss, S. (2004). The prevalence of urinary incontinence in women in four European countries. *BJU International* **93**, 324–330.

Iosif, C. & Bekassy, Z. (1984). Prevalence of genitourinary symptoms in the late menopause. *Acta Obstetricia et Gynecologica Scandinavica* **63**, 257–260.

Jarvis, G. J. (1994). Surgery for stress incontinence. *British Journal of Obstetrics and Gynaecology* **101**, 371–374.

Jolleys, J. V. (1988). Reported prevalence of urinary incontinence in a general practice. *British Medical Journal* **296**, 1300–1302.

Karantanis E, Stanton S, Parsons M, Robinson D, Blackwell AL, Cardozo L, Moore K. (2003). Women's preferences for treatment for stress incontinence – physiotherapy or surgery? *Neurourology and Urodynamics* **22**, 522–523.

Karram, M. M., Yeko, T. R., Sauer, M. V. *et al.* (1989). Urodynamic changes following hormone replacement therapy in women with premature ovarian failure. *Obstetrics and Gynecology* **74**, 208–211.

Kinn, A. C. & Lindskog, M. (1988). Estrogens and phenylpropanolamine in combination for stress urinary incontinence in postmenopausal women. *Urology* **32**, 273–280.

Kondo, A., Kato, K., Saito, M. *et al.* (1990). Prevalence of hand washing incontinence in females in comparison with stress and urge incontinence. *Neurourology and Urodynamics* **9**, 330–331.

Lehtonen T. Rannikko S. Lindell O. Talja M. Wuokko E. Lindskog M. (1986) The effect of phenylpropanolamine on female stress urinary incontinence. *Annales Chirurgiae et Gynaecologiae* **75**, 236–241.

Lin H. H., Sheu, B. C., Lo, M. C. & Huang, S. C. (1999). Comparison of treatment outcomes for imipramine for female genuine stress incontinence. *British Journal of Obstetrics and Gynaecology* **106**, 1089–1092.

Malone-Lee, J. (1988). Urodynamic measurement and urinary incontinence in the elderly. In *Managing and Measuring Incontinence* (ed. J. C. Brocklehurst.). *Proceedings of the Geriatric Workshop on Incontinence, July 1988.*

Millard, R., Moore, K., Yalcin, I. & Bump, R. (2003). Duloxetine vs. placebo in the treatment of stress urinary incontinence: a global phase III study. *Neurourology and Urodynamics* **22**, 482–483.

Moehrer, B., Hextall, A. & Jackson, S. (2003). Oestrogens for urinary incontinence in women. *The Cochrane Database of Systematic Reviews 2003*, issue 2, Article number CD001405. (DOI: 10.1002/14651858.CD001405.)

Norton, P. A., Zinner, N. R., Yalcin, I. & Bump, R. C. (2002). Duloxetine Urinary Incontinence Study Group. Duloxetine versus placebo in the treatment of stress urinary incontinence. *American Journal of Obstetrics and Gynecology* **187**, 40–48.

Park, W. C. & Jordan, V. C. (2002). Selective oestrogen receptor modulators (SERMS) and their roles in cancer prevention. *Trends in Molecular Medicine* **8**, 82–88.

Robinson, D., Cardozo, L., Akeson, M., Hvistendahl, G., Riis, A. & Norgaard, J. P. (2004). Antidiuresis: a new concept in managing female daytime urinary incontinence. *BJU International* **93**, 996–1000.

Rud, T. (1980). The effects of oestrogens and gestagens on the urethral pressure profile in urinary continent and stress incontinent women. *Acta Obstetricia et Gynecologica Scandinavica* **59**, 265–270.

Rud, T., Anderson, K. E., Asmussen, M. *et al.* (1980). Factors maintaining the urethral pressure in women. *Investigative Urology* **17**, 343–347.

Salmon, U. L., Walter, R. I. & Gast, S. H. (1941). The use of oestrogen in the treatment of dysuria and incontinence in postmenopausal women. *American Journal of Obstetrics and Gynecology* **14**, 23–31.

Samsioe, G. (1998). Urogenital ageing – a hidden problem. *American Journal of Obstetrics and Gynecology* **178**, S245–S249.

Samsioe, G., Jansson, I., Mellstrom, D. & Svandborg, A. (1985). Occurence, nature and treatment of urinary incontinence in a 70 year old female population. *Maturitas* **7**, 335–342.

Sandford, J. P. (1975). Urinary tract symptoms and infection. *Annual Review of Medicine* **26**, 485–505.

Shenfield, O. Z., Blackmore, P. F., Morgan, C. W., Schlossberg, S. M., Jordan, G. H. & Ratz, P. H. (1998). Rapid effects of oestriol and progesterone on tone and spontaneous rhythmic contractions of the rabbit bladder. *Neurourology and Urodynamics* **17**, 408–409.

Silfen, S. L., Ciaccia, A. V. & Bryant, H. U. (1999). Selective oestrogen receptor modulators: tissue selectivity and differential uterine effects. *Climacteric* **2**, 268–283.

Smith, P. J. B. (1976). The effect of oestrogens on bladder function in the female. In *The Management of the Menopause and Postmenopausal Years* (ed. S. Campbell), pp. 291–298 Carnforth: MTP.

Thomas, T. M., Plymat, K. R., Blannin, J. *et al.* (1980). Prevalence of urinary incontinence. *British Medical Journal* **281**, 1243–1245.

Thor, K. B. & Katofiasc, M. A. (1995). Effects of duloxetine, a combined serotonin and norepinephrine reuptake inhibitor, on central neural control of lower urinary tract function in the chloralose-anesthetised female cat. *Journal of Pharmacology and Experimental Therapeutics* **274**, 1014–1024.

Van Kerrebroeck, P., Abrams, P., Lange, R., *et al.* (2004). Duloxetine versus placebo in the treatment of European and Canadian women with stress urinary incontinence. *British Journal of Obstetrics and Gynaecology* **111**, 1–9.

Versi, E. & Cardozo, L. D. (1988). Oestrogens and lower urinary tract function. In *The Menopause* (ed. J. W. W. Studd & M. I. Whitehead), pp. 76–84. Oxford: Blackwell Scientific Publications.

Walter, S., Wolf, H., Barlebo, H. & Jansen, H. (1978). Urinary incontinence in postmenopausal women treated with oestrogens: a double-blind clinical trial. *Journal of Urology* **33**, 135–143.

Wilson, P. D., Faragher, B., Butler, B., Bullock, D., Robinson, E. L. & Brown, A. D. G. (1987). Treatment with oral piperazine oestrone sulphate for genuine stress incontinence in postmenopausal women. *British Journal of Obstetrics and Gynaecology* **94**, 568–574.

Youngblood, V. H., Tomlin, E. M. & Davis, J. B. (1957). Senile urethritis in women. *Journal of Urology* **78**, 150–152.

Editors' note (see p.132)

The role of oestrogen replacement therapy in the prevention of ischaemic heart disease has recently been assessed in a 4-year randomized trial, the Heart and Estrogen/progestin Replacement Study (HERS)[i] involving 2763 postmenopausal women younger than 80 yrs with intact uteri and ischaemic heart disease. In the study 55% of women reported at least one episode of urinary incontinence each week, and were randomly assigned to oral conjugated oestrogen plus medroxyprogesterone acetate or placebo daily.

Incontinence improved in 26% of women assigned to placebo as compared to 21% receiving HRT while 27% of the placebo group complained of worsening symptoms compared with 39% in the HRT group ($p = 0.001$). The incidence of incontinent episodes per week increased an average of 0.7 in the HRT group and decreased by 0.1 in the placebo group ($p < 0.001$). Overall combined hormone replacement therapy was associated with worsening stress and urge urinary incontinence although there was no significant difference in daytime frequency, nocturia or number of urinary tract infections.

These findings have also been confirmed in the Nurse's Health Study which followed 39 436 post-menopausal women aged 50–75 years over a four year period The risk of incontinence was found to be elevated in those women taking HRT when compared to those who had never taken HRT. There was an increase in risk in women taking oral oestrogen (RR 1.54; 95% CI 1.44–1.65), transdermal oestrogen (RR 1.68; 95% CI 1.41–2.00), oral oestrogen and progesterone (RR 1.34; 95% CI 1.24–1.34) and transdermal oestrogen and progesterone (RR 1.46; CI 1.16–1.84). In addition, whilst there was remained a small risk after the cessation of HRT (RR 1.14; 95% CI 1.06–1.23) by ten years the risk was identical (RR 1.02; 95% 0.91–1.41) and was identical to those women who had never taken HRT.[ii]

The most recent paper to be reported by the Women's Health Initiative (WHI) writing group has studied the effect of oestrogens with and without progestogens on urinary incontinence.[iii] This paper represents another sub-analysis of the data although it should be remembered that the study was not designed to assess urinary incontinence and thus may lack the appropriate power to do so conclusively.

Overall 27 347 post-menopausal women aged 50 to 79 years were assessed in a multicentre, double blind placebo controlled trial. Of these 23 296 were known to complain of lower urinary tract symptoms at baseline and one year follow up. Women were randomised based on hysterectomy status to active treatment or placebo in either the oestrogen and progestogen or oestrogen only trials. The oestrogen was conjugated equine oestrogen (CEE) whilst the progestogen was medroxyprogesterone acetate (MPA). The main outcome measure was the incidence of urinary incontinence at one year amongst women who were continent at baseline and the severity of urinary incontinence at one year in those who were incontinent at baseline.

Overall hormone replacement therapy was found to increase the incidence of all types of urinary incontinence at one year in those women continent at baseline. The risk was highest for stress incontinence (CEE+MPA; RR 1.87 [1.61–2.18]; CEE alone; RR 2.15 [1.77–2.62]) followed by mixed incontinence (CEE+MPA; RR 1.49 [1.10–2.01]; CEE alone; RR 1.79 [1.26–2.53]). However the effect on urge urinary incontinence was not uniform – (CEE+MPA; RR 1.15 [0.99–1.34]; CEE alone; RR 1.32 [1.10–1.58]).

When considering those women who were symptomatic at baseline urinary frequency was found to increase in both arms (CEE+MPA; RR 1.38 [1.28–1.49]; CEE alone; RR 1.47 [1.35–1.61]) and the incidence of urinary incontinence was seen to increase at one year (CEE+MPA; RR 1.20 [1.06–1.36]; CEE alone; RR 1.59 [1.39–1.82]). In addition, whilst no formal Quality of Life (QoL) assessment was reported, women receiving hormone replacement therapy were more likely to report that urinary incontinence limited their daily activities and bothered and disturbed them.

These results, whilst supportive of the previously reported HERS study and Nurse Health study, would certainly seem to contradict much of the previous work assessing the use of oestrogens in the management of lower urinary tract symptoms.

[i] Grady D, Brown JS, Vittinghoff E, Applegate W, Varner E, Synder T. (2001). Postmenopausal hormones and incontinence: the Heart and Estrogen/progestin Replacement Study. *Obstetrics and Gynaecology* **97**, 116–120.

[ii] Grodstein F, Lifford K, Resnick NM, Curhan GC. (2004). Postmenopausal hormone therapy and risk of developing urinary incontinence. *Obstetrics and Gynaecology* **103**, 254–260.

[iii] Hendrix SL, Cochrane BR, Nygaard IE, Handa VL, Barnabei VM, Iglesia C, Aragaki A, Naughton MJ, Wallace RB, Mc Neeley SG. (2005). Effects of estrogen with and without progestin on urinary incontinence. *JAMA* **293** (8), 935–948.

Chapter 11

The evidence base for surgical intervention in stress urinary incontinence

Gaia Bellini and A. R. B. Smith

Introduction

This review focuses on the assessment of surgical procedures to treat stress urinary incontinence (SUI) in women and analyses the evidence in the medical literature to provide recommendations. Levels of evidence and grades of recommendations are given according with the International Consultation of Urological Diseases (ICUD) system.

Despite the number of operations described to treat stress incontinence and studies conducted, there is no consensus on which of them is most effective. A systematic review of the literature analysed the methodological quality of heterogeneous studies including randomised trials, non-randomised prospective studies and retrospective cohort studies evaluating surgery for stress incontinence and concluded that it was poor (Black & Downes 1996).

Randomised controlled trials (RCTs) provide the most reliable data about the effects of treatments. Subgroup analysis may be useful if there is any risk of different outcome between different treated groups or if there is uncertainty about when to treat (Rothwell 2005). Hilton (2002) confirmed the importance of the studies' population in defining the cure rate of surgical procedures.

Black & Downes (1996) found that non-randomised studies introduced confounder factors such as age, parity, co-morbidity, hormonal status, concomitant or previous surgical procedures. Non-randomised studies also added selection bias which occurred where the choice of surgical procedure was influenced by the patient's anatomy.

The random allocation of treatment may minimise selection bias. Some studies, however, present confounding variables as demonstrated in a randomised trial comparing Burch retropubic urethropexy and anterior colporrhaphy. Confounding factors, such as age, in the two groups, hormonal status, and concurrent surgery in addition to anti-incontinence procedures were included (Kammerer 1999). Other confounding factors are due to the surgeon's technique, skills, equipment and type of anaesthesia as reported by Hilton (2002). This author also emphasised the lack of outcome measures to summarise the effect of treatment. Objective urodynamic outcome measures have been reported in several studies to define cure rate. However, urodynamic measures have no correlation with clinical outcome. Hilton (2002) reported the objective cure rate, based on urodynamic and one hour pad test results, and the subjective cure rate of a randomised trial comparing TVT and colposuspension. Both the procedures resulted in objective cure rates of 81% and 65%, while the subjective cure rate was only 28% and 36% respectively (Hilton 2002; Ward 2002).

The Standardisation Committee of the International Continence Society made recommendations for outcomes of research investigating the effect of therapeutic interventions for women with incontinence. Clinical research must include outcome measures including anatomic and physiologic evaluation, symptoms assessment and objective quantification of symptoms with pad tests and voiding diaries and quality of life measures. Whenever possible, it is also suggested that economic outcomes should be included (Abrams 2002).

Review of procedures

Anterior colporrhaphy

Anterior colporrhaphy is an operation historically used for stress incontinence. It is also a method for treating anterior vaginal prolapse. The vaginal mucosa below the urethra is dissected through a midline incision. A layer of endopelvic fascia is created to support and elevate the bladder neck.

Relatively low cure rates of urinary stress incontinence have been shown by randomised trials.

A long-term prospective randomised study comparing anterior repair and colposuspension was reported and it confirmed the poor medium to long-term results of anterior colporrhaphy when used for stress incontinence. The authors analysed a sample of 71 women undergoing surgery for urodynamic stress incontinence with a follow-up continued for 8 to 17 years. In the group of women having anterior repair, the subjective and objective cure rates were 52% and 42% (Colombo et al. 2000).

Prospective randomised studies reported that the cure rate declined with time. Liapis et al. (1996) showed a cure rate of 75% at 2 months after surgery and 57% after 3 years (level of evidence, 1). Bergman & Elia (1995) found that the objective cure rate dropped from 63% at 1 year follow-up to 37% at the 5 year evaluation (level of evidence, 1). One year follow-up was also evaluated by Kammer et al. (1999) in a randomised trial comparing anterior colporrhaphy and Burch retropubic urethropexy. The authors confirm a low objective cure rate of 31% for women treated with anterior repair. A recent comparative study between anterior colporrhaphy and the Bologna operation for the treatment of anterior wall prolapse associated with stress incontinence after 3 years follow-up concluded that Bologna operation was more effective. The subjective and objective cure rates for the two groups were respectively 57% and 53% for the anterior repair group and 87% and 84% for the Bologna procedure (Tayrak et al. 2002) (level of evidence, 2).

Despite the poor cure rate reported, anterior repair is still used for operative treatment of stress incontinence and concurrent correction of anterior prolapse due to the low morbidity reported.

In a large series of 519 bladder buttress procedures, Beck *et al.* (1991) described serious complication rates of 1% and an incidence of long-term voiding disorders that approached zero. The failure rate associated with *de novo* detrusor overactivity was not higher than 8% (level 2). These data were endorsed by a comparative series between anterior repair and different anti-incontinence procedure when a 5% complication rate at 5 years follow-up was reported (Tamussino *et al.* 1999).

A recent Cochrane review by Glazener and Cooper (Cochrane Database Systematic Review 2004a), analysed literature trials which included anterior vaginal repair in one arm compared with other anti-incontinence procedures. The authors found that important morbidity outcomes, such as voiding dysfunction and detrusor overactivity, were not consistently reported and concluded that they should be incorporated in future research into incontinence. They also confirmed the need of a validated, objective and simple outcome measure for future studies.

Although the cure rate from anterior colporrhaphy appears to be worse than other procedures (level of evidence, 2–3), the lower morbidity associated with the procedure may support its use.

Colposuspension

Colposuspension was first described at the beginning of the 1960's and in some detail by Burch in 1968 and became a reference procedure in the treatment of urodynamic stress incontinence. In the original technique it was performed by suturing the paravaginal fascia, lateral to the bladder neck, to the ileopectineal ligaments bilaterally with three absorbable sutures (Burch 1968). Now, it is commonly performed by placing two to three non-absorbable sutures.

Based on PubMed research, seven RCTs were reviewed (Colombo *et al.* 1996; Colombo *et al.* 2000; Culligan *et al.* 2003; Kammarer-Doak *et al.* 1999; Liapis *et al.* 1996; Wang & Chen 2003; Ward & Hilton 2004). However, comparisons between different trials are difficult due to different techniques used, varied outcome measurements, bias introduced by concomitant procedures, different hormonal status of subgroups, small population sizes and different lengths of follow-up.

In a meta-analysis, the population treated with colposuspension was 341 women versus 344 who had other surgical procedures. The mean age was 53.8 (36–75). The cure rates were defined as objective or subjective, but they were determined on the basis of different parameters by different authors (Table 11.1) and both were not always reported. The mean objective cure rate was 80.4% (51–100) and the mean subjective cure rate reported in six studies was 84% (37–100) at a follow up from 1 year to 17 years.

Table 11.1 Summary of randomised controlled trials on Burch colposuspension versus other procedures for the treatment of urodynamic stress incontinence in women: main criteria

Authors	Total number of women	Number of women in Burch arm	Follow-up length	Per cent OBJ cure rate	Per cent SUBJ cure rate	OBJ assessment	SUBJ assessment	Complications (%)	Level of evidence
Colombo et al. (2000)	71	35	2.7 years (9–17)	74	86	Negative stress test	History	Recurrent cystocele (33)	2
Colombo et al. (1996)	36	18	2.2 years (1–3)	100	100	Negative stress test	History	Persistent voiding difficulties (17)	2
Liapis et al. (1996)	81	41	3 years	88	Not reported	Negative cough profile	—	None	2
Ward & Hilton (2004)	344	169	2 years	51	20 (no leakage) 37 (patient report of "cure")	1 h pad-test ≤ 1 g	BFLUTS questionnaire: No leakage Or patient's report of "cure"	-Persistent voiding difficulties (2.7) -Wound infection (7)	1
Wang & Chen (2003)	90	41	22 months (12–36)	76	93	1 h pad-test ≤ 2 g	No loss urine during exercise	Voiding difficulties	2
Kammarer-Doak et al. (1999)	35	18	1 year	83	93	Negative cough test + valsalva manoeuvre (supine & standing positions)	Subjective rate of symptoms	none	2
Culligan (2003)	36	19	72.6 months (33–116)	84.6	93	Negative cough test + valsalva manoeuvre (supine and standing position)	No leakage episodes on 24h voiding diary	none	2

The mechanism through which colposuspension procedures restore continence is still debated. It has been suggested that a mechanical action elevates the bladder neck and compresses the urethra against the anterior vaginal wall when an increase in abdominal pressure occurs (Bombieri *et al.* 2002a). Recently Digesu *et al.* (2004) used magnetic resonance imaging to study the levator ani muscle position in relation with the bladder neck after colposuspension and found that surgical success was significantly associated with a shorter distance between the two. Objective cure rate was 86% (24 of 28 women studied) at one year follow-up (level of evidence, 2).

Pre- and postoperative urodynamic studies were reviewed in 88 patients who had a colposuspension by Dolan *et al.* (2004) in a retrospective cohort study that suggested the relevance of sub-urethral support. They found that, postoperatively, opening detrusor pressure increased only in women who were objectively cured after the procedure and that it was significantly higher in younger patients. The objective cure rate was 69% (level of evidence, 3).

Long-term follow up results have been reported by several authors and postoperative complications have been described. Langer *et al.* (2001) followed up 127 patients for 10–15 years (mean 12.5) and reported an objective cure rate of 93.7%. They described postoperative complications such as detrusor overactivity (16.6%) within the first postoperative year and anatomical defects (18.7%) that were detected in most after five years (level of evidence, 3). In a longitudinal retrospective study of 109 patients with a mean follow-up of 13.8 years (10–20) treated with primary or secondary colposuspension, Alcalay *et al.* (1995) described a drop in the cure rate that reached a plateau of 69% after 10–12 years. They reported 14.5% and 15.1% of postoperative detrusor overactivity after primary and secondary colposuspension respectively, 4.6% of recurrent urinary tract infections and 22% of voiding difficulties. Urethotomies were performed in 3.7% women for persistent voiding difficulties (level of evidence, 3). Similarly, a recent prospective cohort study found 3.5% of persistent voiding dysfunctions after colposuspension performed in 310 women with a mean follow-up of 36 months (Vierek *et al.* 2004) (level of evidence, 2). A population of 77 women was studied by Bombieri *et al.* (2002b) with magnetic resonance imaging the day before surgery and six days after the procedure and urodynamic investigations preoperatively and three months after colposuspension. They found that bladder neck elevation and anterior compression of the urethra were significantly associated with detrusor overactivity at three months (21.4% *de novo* detrusor overactivity reported) and with the number of days of catheterisation. They described 7.7% of voiding dysfunctions at three months follow-up and 2.5% at one year (level of evidence, 2). Maher *et al.* (1999) reported 4% voiding difficulties as requiring intermittent self-catheterisation for at least four months in a series of 53 women after colposuspension for recurrent urodynamic stress incontinence following retropubic procedures. The postoperative subjective cure rate was 80% and the objective cure rate was 72%. Postoperative detrusor overactivity was found in 6% of patients (level of evidence, 3). Successful results for Burch colposuspension as secondary procedure were also reported by Thakar *et al.* (2002). She reviewed 56 women with a mean follow up of four years and found a subjective cure rate of 71% and objective cure rate of 80% (level of evidence, 2).

Dwyer *et al.* (1999) described two cases of non-absorbable suture into the bladder following colposuspension presenting with frequency and dysuria in a series of 1103 colposuspension performed.

By elevating the anterior vaginal wall and altering the vaginal axis, Burch colposuspension may predispose to posterior and upper anatomical defects. Kwon *et al.* (2003) examined 36 of 60 women after colposuspension without symptomatic , POP-Q) prolapse. Only one patient required surgery (level of evidence, 3).

In summary, the evidence available illustrates the effectiveness of open colposuspension for the treatment of SUI (level 1) with medium term follow-up as a primary or secondary procedure. No higher morbidity or complications were found when compared with other anti-incontinence procedures (level 1). Voiding dysfunction, utero-vaginal prolapse and detrusor overactivity were the main complications related to the procedure (level 1).

Open colposuspension can be recommended as an effective procedure for stress incontinence of urine (Grade A).

Laparoscopic colposuspension

Laparoscopic colposuspension was first described by Vancaille in 1991 (Vancaille 1991). Since then it has become popular because of the potential advantages of a minimal access procedure such as smaller incision, minimal blood loss, reduced duration of hospital stay and length of convalescence when compared with open colposuspension.

Six randomised trials comparing laparoscopic and open colposuspension have been reported in the literature (Ankardal *et al.* 2004). Moherer (2004) fully analysed five of them in a systematic Cochrane review (Burton 1997; Carey *et al.* 2000; Fatthy *et* al. 2001; Summitt *et al.* 2000; Su *et al.* 1997) that concluded that the laparoscopic approach was associated with a lower cure rate. Three of the randomised trials were only reported as abstracts (Burton 1997; Carey *et al.* 2000; Summitt *et al.* 2000) and unpublished information was obtained by interviewing the authors. At a follow-up of 6–18 months, subjective cure rate ranged from 85–96% and 85–100% in the laparoscopic and in the open groups respectively, when four RCTs were included. Burton's study was excluded because data were reported as visual analogical scale results. However, Su's study was then excluded too because there were problems with randomisation and different use of suture: one suture for laparoscopic colposuspension and three sutures for the open procedure. There was a non significant increase of cure rate for the laparoscopic arm (5% higher cure rate; relative risk (RR) 1.05, 95% confidence interval (CI) 0.99–1.11). Objective cure rate assessed with urodynamic evaluation was significantly higher after open procedure in all five studies (RR 0.89, 95% CI 0.82–0.98) with an addition of 9% risk of failure after laparoscopic surgery. When Su's study was excluded, the difference in cure rate was not significant (RR 0.91, 95% CI 0.82–1.01). Moehrer underlined the importance of the experience of the surgeon in the success rate of the laparoscopic procedure and noted Burton's inexperience in performing laparoscopic colposuspension when commencing the trial. Other possible biases were different types and number of sutures used by different authors.

Although surgical outcome analysis revealed higher peri-operative complications among laparoscopic procedures, for example bladder injuries and cases of laceration to the obturator vein, the difference was not significant (RR 1.16, 95% CI 0.59–2.29; Burton 1997; Carey *et al.* 2000; Fatthy *et* al. 2001; Summitt *et al.* 2000; Su *et al.* 1997). Higher postoperative morbidity was found for open colposuspension when compared with laparoscopic procedure, as was longer hospital stay and return to normal activities, higher blood loss (Burton 1997; Carey *et al.* 2000; Fatthy *et* al. 2001; Summitt *et al.* 2000; Su *et al.* 1997) and longer catheterisation (Burton 1997; Carey *et al.* 2000; Su *et al.* 1997). Laparoscopic colposuspension required less analgesia and patients complained about less pain but quantitative analysis was not presented (Burton 1997; Carey *et al.* 2000; Fatthy *et* al. 2001; Su *et al.* 1997). Operative time was longer for laparoscopic surgery in four trials (Burton 1997; Carey *et al.* 2000; Fatthy *et* al. 2001; Summitt *et al.* 2000).

A recent randomised trial that compared open colposuspension using suturing with laparoscopic surgery using mesh showed objective and subjective cure rates at one year follow-up higher for open colposuspension (92% and 89% for open colposuspension versus 74% and 62% for laparoscopic surgery, $p < 0.001$) with less peri-operative time, but significantly longer catheterisation time ($p < 0.01$), greater risk of urinary retention ($p < 0.01$), more blood loss ($p < 0.0001$) and a longer hospital stay ($p < 0.0001$). Complications described, equally presented in both laparoscopic and open arms, were bladder perforation, urinary tract infection and wound infection. One case of haematoma leading to re-operation was described in the laparoscopic group (Ankardal *et al.* 2004). In a retrospective comparative study, Saidi *et al.* (1998) found similar short-term cure rates and complication rates when 70 laparoscopic colposuspensions were compared with 87 open procedures (91.4 versus 92%, and 15.8% versus 33.3%, respectively).

Other authors described complications such as ureteric ligation with the suture (Dwyen *et al.* 1999, Asloan *et al.* 1997), urinary tract injury, bowel injury, vessel injury, important blood loss and abscess formation in Retzius' space that were reported in 25% of cases by Paraiso *et al.* (1999). Only one randomised trial by Persson *et al.* (2004) that compared different methods of laparoscopic colposuspension was reported by Moherer *et al.* (2004) in the Cochrane review. It compared one single suture with double suture and found that the objective and subjective cure rates were 65% and 58% versus 89% and 83% respectively.

Complications described were pubis osteitis in the one suture group, recurrent stress incontinence that required reoperation in the two sutures group, postoperative urge symptoms and voiding dysfunction in both groups.

In an attempt to decrease the operating time, different laparoscopic techniques using mesh, tacks and clips have been introduced. In a randomised trial of 60 women, Zullo *et al.* (2001) compared the transperitoneal technique using non-absorbable sutures with Prolene mesh fixed with tacks or staples and found that the objective failure rate was significantly lower in the first group at 1 year follow-up (11.1% versus 26.9%, $p < 0.05$). Kenton *et al.* (2002) reported two cases of multiple foreign body perforation into the bladder following a laparoscopic colposuspension modified by the use of mesh.

In summary, even though open Burch colposuspension seemed to achieve a higher cure rate than laparoscopic procedure (level of evidence, 1–2), the studies reported only short-term follow-up of poor quality data and sometimes by inexperienced surgeons. Long-term follow-up of randomised trials by skilled surgeons is required to determine whether laparoscopic colposuspension can be recommended as an alternative to open colposuspension.

Paravaginal repair

Paravaginal defects were first described by White in 1909 who demonstrated that cystoceles were caused by a detachment of the anterior endopelvic fascia from its lateral attachment to the arcus tendineus fascia pelvis and suggested the vaginal paravaginal repair for the correction of cystoceles (White 1909).

The paravaginal repair procedure re-attaches the lateral vaginal wall to the arcus tendineus fascia pelvis and is used in women with stress incontinence and lateral anterior vaginal wall defects. It can be performed vaginally, abdominally or laparoscopically through the Retzius space.

Only one randomised controlled trial comparing paravaginal repair with colposuspension has been reported. The authors randomised 36 women at the time of surgery and reported follow-up after one and three years. The objective and subjective cure rate for colposuspension and paravaginal repair were 100% and 72% versus 100% and 61%, respectively. The authors concluded that paravaginal repair is less effective than colposuspension in treating stress incontinence, but resumption of voiding was achieved earlier in the paravaginal repair group. One woman who had colposuspension developed detrusor overactivity, but none occurred in the paravaginal repair group (Colombo *et al.* 1996) (level of evidence, 1–2).

Similar results were reported in a small study by Mallipeddi *et al.* (2001). The authors recruited 45 women with bilateral paravaginal support defects (21 of whom presented with urodynamic stress incontinence) and a vaginal paravaginal repair was performed. The outcome was assessed by IIQ/UDI questionnaire, vaginal evaluation, voiding diary and standing stress test. Long-term follow-up of minimum

Table 11.2 Summary of studies on laparoscopic colposuspension for the treatment of urodynamic stress incontinence in women. Main criteria

Authors	Number of women	Follow-up length	Per cent OBJ cure rate	Per cent SUBJ cure rate	OBJ cure rate criteria	SUBJ cure rate criteria	Operating time (min) (mean (SD))	Estimated blood loss (ml) (mean (SD))	Hospital stay (days) Mean (SD)	Catheterisation length (days) (mean (SD))	Level of evidence
Ankardal et al. (2004); RCT	#LC 109 (105) ##OBC 109 (97)	1 year	74 92	62 89	48 h voiding diary + 48 h pad-test	Subjective assessment	75 (24) 60 (19)	35 (101) 105 (99)	$2.2 (1.3) $3.9 (1.5)	1.9 (2.4) 4.9 (8.3)	1-2
Carey et al. (2001); RCT	LC 104 OBC 96	6 months	69 80	100 95	Urodynamics	Subjective success	85 44	125 171	3.7 3.9	4.4 4.9	1-2
Fatty et al. (2001); RCT	LC 34 OBC 40	1.5 years	88 85	—	Urodynamics	—	70.18 (16.54) 53 (10.05)	42.75 (7.2) 240.5(35.5)	1.5 (0.25) 3.18(0.42)	—	1-2
Summitt et al. (2000); RCT	LC 62 OBC 28	1 year	93 88	—	Urodynamics	—	173.2 118.6	112 131.9	1.4 2.1	2.7 2.7	1-2
Burton (1997); RCT	LC 30 OC 30	5 years	57 90	—	voiding diary + 1 h pad-test + urodynamics+ VCUG	—	°°83 (74–110) °°42 (35–52)	°°190 (180–290) °°261 (120–410)	2.8 4.16	1.33 1.7	1-2
Su et al. (1997); RCT	LC 46* OBC 46**	1 year	80 96	—	Urodynamic evaluations	—	66.5 (15.5) 72.8 (23.5)	59.3 (42.1) 134.3 (102)	3.93 5.15	3.9 (1.9) 6.8 (2.3)	1-2
Persson et al. (2000); RCT	LC one stitch: 78 LC two stitches: 83	1 year (median)	83 58	65 85	Ultrashort pad-test	questionnaire	°°60 (35–121) °°77 (45–110)	15 16	°°1.7 °°1.7	—	1-2
Zullo et al. (2001); RCT	LC nas 30 (A) LC prolene mesh+staples 30 (B)	12	**Failure rates** SUBJ: A=7.4; B=15.4; OBJ: A=11.1; B=26.9		Urodynamics	Visual analog scale of leakage	67.9±7.5 62.1±4.8	A= 118±76 B=130±91	A=1.7±1.3 B=1.6±1.4 (postoperative H. stay)	—	2

LC, laparoscopic colposuspension; LC nas, laparoscopic colposuspension using not absorbable suture; OBC, open Burch colposuspension; OBJ, objective; SUBJ, subjective; VCUG, videocystourethrography; *, one stitch; **, two stitches; #, laparoscopic mesh colposuspension; ##, open Burch colposuspension using stitches; $, nights; °°, median + range values.

of one year to maximum of 2.8 years was achieved for 35 patients. The recurrence rate of cystocele, enterocele and rectocele were 3%, 20% and 14% respectively. Persistent stress incontinence was found in 57% of women. One case of intraoperative complication was described as bilateral ureteric obstruction. Postoperative morbidity included one retropubic haematoma which needed re-exploration and two cases of vaginal abscesses (level of evidence, 3–4).

Shull *et al.* reported a larger study which included 149 women who suffered from stress incontinence and cystocele that were treated by paravaginal repair with 6 years follow-up. Postoperatively, 6% and 5% of patients developed respectively cuff prolapse and enterocele. In 5% there was a persistent cystocele. The incontinence cure rate was 97% (Shull *et al.* 1989, level of evidence, 4).

Ostrzenski *et al.* (1998) performed laparoscopic paravaginal repair in 28 women with stress incontinence and anterior lateral vaginal defects. All of them achieved a follow-up of three months and one year and were assessed by clinical examination, voiding diary, stress test and urodynamic pre- and postoperatively. The authors reported a cure rate of 93% (level of evidence, 4).

The laparoscopic approach is also described by Miklos *et al.* (2002) who performed paravaginal repair combined with Burch urethropexy in 130 of a series of 170 women with paravaginal defects and stress incontinence. He recorded four cystotomies during the procedures.

Scotti *et al.* (1998) reported a cure rate from stress incontinence at a mean of 39 months follow-up of 94.4% in 36 of 40 patients that he treated with paravaginal repair for paravaginal defects and stress incontinence. However, he combined paravaginal repair with other procedures such as Burch or suburethral sling urethropexy to correct urethral hypermobility that he detected with 'cotton swab test'.

In conclusion, only one randomised trial has compared paravaginal repair with open colposuspension for the treatment of SUI. This study concluded that paravaginal repair is less effective (level of evidence, 2). Other level 3 studies have also suggested lower cure rates with paravaginal repair. Only when combined with other anti-incontinence operations was the cure rate higher (level of evidence, 3–4).

Marshall–Marchetti–Krantz procedure

The Marshall–Marchetti–Krantz (MMK) procedure is one variation of open retropubic colposuspension and it consists of suspension of the bladder neck onto the periosteum or cartilage of the symphysis pubis.

Two randomised trials have compared the MMK procedure to the Burch colposuspension, but the numbers studied were small, the objective and subjective cure rate definitions were different (Quadri *et al.* 1999; Colombo *et al.* 1994) and Colombo *et al.* used a modified MMK technique by opening the anterior bladder wall. In the latter study, 80 patients were randomised into the two surgical procedures and had a mean follow-up of 3.5 and 3.1 years (range 2–7 years) for the MMK and the Burch colposuspension groups, respectively. Although the difference for the objective and the subjective cure rates was not statistically significant between the two, (80% and 92% versus 65% and 85% respectively), resumption of voiding took longer in the MMK arm. This finding was also described by Quadri *et al.* (1999). They reported an objective cure rate of 93% and a subjective cure rate of 100% for 15 women treated with MMK at one year follow-up. Both authors recognised one case of retropubic hematoma following the MMK procedure and Colombo *et al.* also described one case of recurrent stress incontinence, one case of severe voiding difficulty and four cases of *de novo* detrusor overactivity in the same group.

Osteitis pubis was described by Kammerer *et al.* (1998) in 0.74% of 2030 MMK urethropexy procedures performed from 1980 to 1994. The mean time of onset of symptoms was 69.8 days postoperatively (range 10 to 459 days). A review of 56 mainly retrospective studies reported an incidence of 1–2.5% of the same complication. The articles included 2712 cases and the overall success rate was 86.1% (92.1% for primary procedures and 21.1% for repeat procedures. The mean complication rate reported was 21.1%) (Mainprize *et al.* 1988).

Long-term results are described in only a few articles which mainly reported subjective cure rates obtained by questionnaire or telephone interviews. The success rate decreased with time in a retrospective study of 60 women followed up at 6, 12, 60 and 120 months postoperative and was 81%, 77%, 57% and 28% respectively (Czapliki *et al.* 1998, level 3). Clemens *et al.* (1998) found that the subjective cure rate in 36 of 56 patients previously treated with the MMK procedure was 33% at a mean follow-up of 16.8 years (range 13.2–21.9). Hegarty *et al.* (2001) described the subjective cure rate in 40 women and it was 82% postoperative and 61% at a mean follow-up of 8.5 years. All failures occurred within 2 years of the operations.

Although there is some evidence to suggest similar cure rates between Marshall-Marchetti-Krantz and open Burch colposuspension (level 2–3), osteitis pubis described in many retrospective studies (level 3) limits the value of the procedure.

Needle suspension

Needle suspension may be performed from an abdominal or a vaginal approach. A needle is passed through the cave of Retzius space blindly to thread sutures from the vagina to the anterior abdominal fascia, on each side of the bladder neck. There are several types and modifications of the first procedure described by Pereyra (1959) such as Stamey (1973), Raz (1981) and Gittes & Loughlin (1987), dependant on the type, numbers and site of attachment of the sutures.

To provide evidence of the short and long-term effectiveness of needle suspension procedures, Glazener and Cooper reviewed nine randomised or quasi-randomised trials that included 347 women treated with needle suspension and 437 treated with other procedures (Glazener & Cooper 2004b). Four of the studies included women with primary urodynamic stress incontinence and five included either primary or recurrent urodynamic stress incontinence. Four small studies compared needle suspension to colposuspension as secondary anti-incontinence procedure and found no difference between the two procedures.

When compared with colposuspension in seven trials, the subjective success rate was significantly inferior (71% versus 84% at one year follow up), but there was no difference in peri-operative complications (23% versus 16%). There was no significant difference in other outcome measures.

Two trials compared needle suspension with anterior colporrhaphy and the subjective cure rate was similar (65% versus 62%), both in women with or without prolapse.

Long-term results, reported from a RCT and subsequent five years follow-up, showed that the efficacy of needle suspension decreased with time and subjective cure rate was 72% and 43% at one year and five years respectively (Bergman et al. 1989; Bergman et al. 1995). In a recent retrospective study, Gilja et al. (2000) reported the same trend describing a decrease of the subjective cure rate from the six months to the 1–5 years follow-up, 92%, and 76% respectively (level 3). Other studies have shown similar results. Masson et al. (2000) retrospectively considered charts and video-urodynamic reports of 208 patients who had a modified Pereyra procedure and through questionnaires followed-up 135 women, with a mean follow-up of 4.14 years. Although 69% were satisfied and an improvement was reported in 79%, only 14% reported no leakage. When pre-operative video-urodynamic diagnosis of intrinsic sphincter deficiency was considered, only 2.6% of women were dry, while the outcome was better for women in whom pure bladder neck hypermobility was found: 20% of patients were dry (level 3). Other recent studies are reported in Table 11.3. However, the data are difficult to interpret because in many studies concomitant pelvic floor procedures were performed and patients had SUI alone or with detrusor overactivity. Complications referred both to anti-incontinence procedure alone and to concomitant surgery when performed and primary or secondary procedures were not differentiated (level of evidence, 3).

A modified technique of needle suspension using bone anchors has been reported, but poor results and high incidence of complications were described. Tebyani et al. (2000) followed up 42 of 49 patients who had this procedure with telephone interview at a mean of 29 months (range 16–52) and only 5% of them were subjectively cured. 12% reported an improvement while the failure rate was 83%. One case of osteomyelitis was described and in two patients the bone anchor became detached and migrated into the pelvis. Tsivian et al. (2003) also reported on the use of bone anchors and described complications in eight women in a group of 31. They also reported one case of osteomyelitis, five cases in whom 11 sutures passed through the bladder and only five of them were detected intra-operatively and one case of a vesico-vaginal fistula.

A prospective study described a modified technique that fixed the suspending sutures to Cooper's ligaments. Even though the sample was small (5 of 19 women lost to long-term follow up), the objective cure of 85% at a mean follow-up of 50 months suggested a good outcome (Klutke *et al.* 2000) (level 3).

In conclusion, the higher failure rate without a significant reduction in complications, indicates that needle procedures should no longer be recommended for treatment of stress incontinence of urine.

Pubo-vaginal sling

Pubo-vaginal slings were first described over 100 years ago for the treatment of stress incontinence. Since then, many techniques using different materials have been described, but it is not clear whether they influence the outcome.

One of the most common choices for the sling material is autologous rectus sheath fascia, first described by Aldridge in 1942 (Aldridge 1942). Other organic materials described can be autologous (fascia, tendon, dermis), allografts from human cadavers (fascia, dermis, dura) and xenografts (porcine or bovine dermis, bovine pericardium or intestinal submucosa). Whatever material is used for the sling, it is conventionally positioned under the urethra at the level of the bladder neck. The sling is normally attached to the rectus sheath fascia, but variations of the technique have been described such as Cooper's ligaments or pubis symphysis fixation.

Autologous materials

Rectus sheath fascia and fascia lata slings appear to have some common properties; they are not rejected but their properties vary in different patients. Furthermore, there are few data on the biological process that occurs when they are inserted. Fitzgerald *et al.* (2000) described the histological appearance of autologous rectus fascia obtained by biopsies during postoperative revisions in five patients at 3, 5, 8, 17 weeks and 4 years after the insertions. In all cases, fibroblast proliferation was noticed with different orientations, remodelling of the graft and neovascularisation. No inflammatory reaction or immune responses were seen. However, the authors could not extrapolate the data to successful procedures because the number of patients examined was too small and all of them had recurrent stress incontinence.

The cure rate of SUI following autologous sling has been reported with a range of 84–98% (Beck *et al.* 1988; Chou *et al.* 2003; Hassouna & Ghonhiem 1999; Richter *et al.* 2001).

Common complications have been described, such as the significant time interval from surgery to successful voiding, voiding dysfunction symptoms and *de novo* urge incontinence. In a large series of 170 patients treated with fascia lata graft, Beck *et al.* (1988) reported a mean interval time of 59.6 days after the procedure to successful voiding with 3% undergoing sling release for retention. Richter *et al.* (2001) reported an incidence of 41% post-voiding dysfunction in a sample of 57 patients treated with

Table 11.3 Summary of studies on needle suspension for the treatment of urodynamic stress incontinence in women: main criteria

Authors	Type of study	Number of patients	Follow-up	Per cent OBJ cure rate	Per cent SUBJ cure rate	OBJ criteria	SUBJ criteria	Complications	Level of evidence
Wennberg et al. (2003)	POS	24	63 months (28–100)	42	83	Quantitative evaluation+ Urodynamic results	questionnaire	21% urgency symptoms	3
Takahaski et al. (2002)	RS	86	37.6 months			Complications 37.2%: Voiding difficulties (15) Lower abdominal pain (15) Stitches removed (2)			3
Hutchings & Black (2001)	NRT	54 needle suspension 221 colposuspension 130 anterior colporrhaphies	12 months	13 34 19	68 75 55	Activity daily score	Women's report of improvement	****	3
Tebyani et al. (2000)	RS	49 bone anchors	29 months (16–52)	–	5 cured 12 improved	–	Telephone interview	1 osteomyelitis 2 bone anchors dislodged	3
Gilja (2000)	POS	88 (71 evaluated at 5 years)	5 years	69	76	Clinical evaluation + urodynamic assessment	questionnaire	Unilateral suture removal due to infection 3.4% Inguinal nerve entrapment 2.2% Recurrent SUI 22% De novo urge incontinence 3.4%	3
Tsivian et al. (2003)	POS	31 bone anchors (28 evaluated at 60 months)	67.7 months (60–76)	21.4	–	No pad used	–	11 sutures through the bladder 12 bone anchors dislodged 1 osteomyelitis 1 fistula	3

POS, prospective observational study; RS, retrospective study; NRT, non-randomised trial.

Table 11.3 Continued

Authors	Type of study	Number of patients	Follow-up	Per cent OBJ cure rate	Per cent SUBJ cure rate	OBJ criteria	SUBJ criteria	Complications	Level of evidence
Costantini et al. (2003)	POS	4 corners suspension A = 27urinary incontinence+ cystocoele (14 USI + DO) B=5 urethrocoele repair 5 rectocoele repair	62 months (36–83)	—	85	—	Symptoms	32% urinary retention 50% persistent DO 5% suprapubic haematoma 5% vaginal bleeding 2% vaginal granuloma	3
Nguyen & Bhatia (2001)	RS	A = 34 modified Pereyra B = 28 modified Pereyra + sacrospinous fixation	23 ± 14.4 months	A = 88 B = 61	A = 91 B = 64	No Urodynamic Stress Incontinence at customary	No subjective leakage	Total 18% de novo DO 11% urinary infection Group B 2% transfusion 2%recurrent prolapse 3%gluteal pain	3
Klutke et al. (2000)	POS	19 Cooper's ligaments fixation (14 reviewed)	50 months	86		Stress test at cyst metric capacity		5% de novo DO	3
Hilton & Mayne (1991)	UOS	100 (89 previous anti-incontinence procedures)	27 months (3–51)	<65 years = 53 >65 years = 76 USI + DO preop = 33			Symptoms	1 blood loss >200 ml 3 post-op urinary infection 1 thrombophlebitis 1 deep venous thrombosis 6 pain in suprapubic incision 1 suture passed transvaginally	3

POS, prospective observational study; RS, retrospective study; NRT, non-randomised trial; UOS, uncontrolled observational study.

autologous slings, but other studies have described a lower incidence. Chaikin *et al.* (1998) reported a 2% incidence of permanent urinary retention. McLennan *et al.* (1998) reported a mean of 10 days to resumption of normal voiding and an incidence of 5% of permanent retention in 62 women who underwent fascia lata suburethral sling operations. The authors found that age over 65 years, additional surgical procedures and pre-operative low peak flow rates were risk factors for delayed voiding. The incidence of *de novo* urge incontinence after autologous suburethral slings has been reported as 15–20% (Cross *et al.* 1998; Richter *et al.* 2001; Enzelberger *et al.* 1996). This may be related to bladder outlet obstruction caused by the sling. However, Chou *et al.* (2003) reported a successful cure rate in patients with mixed urinary incontinence of 93% versus 97% for stress incontinence alone; the difference was not statistically significant.

Other rare complications such as urethral erosion have been reported using autologous fascial slings (Golomb *et al.* 2001; Leach *et al.* 1997). Three cases of urethro-vaginal fistula were reported in early experience with fascia lata slings (Bergman & Creder 1997).

The formation of seromas and leg pain are complications described only when a fascia lata sling was used (Beck *et al.* 1988).

Even though long-term data (level 3 or 4) suggest a successful outcome with autologous fascia lata sling procedures (Table 11.4), they require a larger incision and additional surgery to harvest the fascia which increases the peri-operative morbidity, operative time, postoperative pain and hospital stay.

Allografts

In 1996, Handa *et al.* reported preliminary results from the use of allograft fascia lata for suburethral slings (Handa *et al.* 1996) supported by long-term experience in orthopaedic surgery that supported safety, lack of antigenicity and long-term stability (Cooper & Beck 1993). The main perceived advantage is reduced morbidity and postoperative pain, simplification of the operation and an improvement in cosmesis when compared with allograft slings. In addition, there is a decrease in the risk of local complications such as erosion, sinus tract and fistula formation and chronic wound infections when compared with synthetic slings.

Allografts are obtained from cadaveric donors and processed from licensed tissue banks with different techniques such as freezing, freeze-drying or gamma irradiation. Although the risk of transmission of virus infections, such as hepatitis and human immunodeficiency virus, is reduced by multi-step sterilisation processes and serologic screening, and has been estimated as one in eight million (Handa *et al.* 1996), the theoretical risk of transmission of prions still exists. The literature reported 150 cases of iatrogenic Creutzfelt-Jacob disease from transplanted corneas, human growth factors and gonadotrophins derived from cadaveric pituitaries and dura mater grafts prior 1987. However, after 1987 the use of sodium hydroxide in the process of

Table 11.4 Summary of studies on autologous grafts for the treatment of urodynamic stress incontinence in women: main criteria

Authors	Length of sling (cm)	Number of Patients	Mean follow-up (months)	Per cent cure rate of SUI	Per cent persistent storage symptoms	Per cent de novo storage symptoms	Per cent voiding dysfunction
				Rectus Fascia slings			
Groutz et al. (2001)	15	67	34 (12–60)	67.2	—	10	22 weak stream, straining, postural change (SUBJ)
Morgan (2000)	6–8	247 (235 replied to the questionnaire)	51 (22–68)	82.2	26	7	2 urethrolysis for retention >3 months
Jeffrey et al. (2000)	—	35	°39 (30–48)	91.4	5.7	5.7	—
Hassouna & Ghoniem (1999)	7	82	41 (6–96)	49.3 (dry) 89.1 improved	25.9 (of 77 replied on urge incontinence questions)	20.8 (of 77 replied on urge incontinence questions)	—
Kane et al. (1999)	5	13	°26 (19–38)	100	0	8	8 dilation
Barrington et al. (1998)	20	§51 S 22 P	24 (6–48)	94 S 78 P	22 urge symptoms	—	16 persistent high residual volume
Chaikin et al. (1998)	15	251	°37 (12–180)	73 cured 19 improved	41	3	2 permanent urinary retention
Loughlin (1996)	5	22	15 (4–22)	73 cured 18 improved	9	4	23 dilation for transient retention
Mason & Roach (1996)	4	63	15 (4–22)	93.7	—	16 urge incontinence	3 CICS; 2 surgical revision; 2 resuming voiding>7.5 m
Zaragosa (1996)	6–8	60	25 (11–34)	95	31 urgency	12	—

Table 11.4 Continued

Authors	Length of sling (cm)	Number of Patients	Mean follow-up (months)	Per cent cure rate of SUI	Per cent persistent storage symptoms	Per cent de novo storage symptoms	Per cent voiding dysfunction
				Rectus Fascia or Fascia Lata slings			
Flynn (2002)	12	71	44 (30–56)	90.1	28	5	3 Retention> 45 days 1 urethrolysis
Richter (2001)	24	57	42 (0.5–134)	84	18	—	16 persistent high residual volume; postural change 4; CIC 7
Golomb (1997)	15	18	30.7 (12–53)	88.9	0	5 refractory urge 6	—
Haab et al. (1997a)	12–15	37	48.2 (24–60)	73	40	18	CIC 8; refractory urge 24
Kreder (1996)	—	27	22 (9–32)	96.3	63	12	CIC 7
				Fascia Lata slings			
Latini et al. (2004)	18–22	100	52 (8–111)	85 cured or improved	—	—	—
Govier (1997)	24–28	32 (30 telephone Interview)	°14 (3–33)	33 cured 37 improved	18	14	CICS> 3 months 3; sling incision 3
Mc Lennan et al. (1998)	15–20	62	Not mentioned	87	—	—	Urinary retention with sling incision 5
Breen et al. (1997)	15–20	60	12 (6–24)	90 + 3#	33	—	Urinary retention with sling release 13.4
Karram et al. (1990)	5–7	10	12–24	90	10	10	—
Beck (1988)	—	170	1.5–24	98.2	—	—	Mean time to successful voiding 59.6 days; Sling release 3

°CICS, intermittent self catheterisation; CIC, intermittent catheterisation; § S, secondary procedure following previous surgery; P, primary procedure; °, median value; #, 3% slings removed during drainage of postoperative retroperitoneal abscess.

decontamination has reduced the risk of prion infection that is estimated as 1 in 3,500,000 (Amundsen *et al.* 2000).

Fitzgerald *et al.* initially reported an early 22% failure rate when freeze-dried irradiated cadaveric fascia lata was used; they re-operated on 8 of 35 women and described autolysis in seven grafts at the time of re-operation (Fitzgerald *et al.* 1999). Amundsen *et al.* (2000) followed up 91 of 104 women treated with freeze-dried fascia lata for a mean period of 19.4 months and reported an objective cure rate of 63% and improvement (less then 1 pad/day) of 21%; subjective cure rate was 87%. Urge incontinence previously detected in 59 patients resolved in 41% of them. However, they described 15% *de novo* detrusor overactivity which they related to the high incidence of previous pelvic surgery (80%) and previous anti-incontinence procedures (49%). They also reported one case of failure that needed re-operation and one urinary retention treated with urethrolysis. In a smaller study, 26 patients were evaluated with a mean follow-up of 15 months using pad-score and questionnaire. The objective cure rate was 77% and the incidence of improvement, less than one pad/day, was 15.4%; the subjective cure rate was 96%. In two cases, patients described *de novo* urgency symptoms (Elliot & Boone 2000). Cadaveric fascia was processed differently from that of Fitzgerald's study using solvent dehydration instead of freeze-dried specimens. Lemer *et al.* (1999) previously found that consistency of freeze-dried cadaveric fascia is lower than solvent dehydration specimens that otherwise are similar to the autologous tissues. These findings may influence the results.

Other recent studies are reported in Table 11.5 (level of evidence, 2–3) that showed good short and medium term results with a low incidence of complications. However, long-term follow-up is required to determine the rate of complications including failure, infection, disease transmission and sling rejection.

Xenografts

Animal tissues have been employed by several authors for sling operations since 1985. Porcine dermis bladder slings were initially used (Zenoderm, Ethicon) and to prevent rejections the grafts were cross linked with aldehyde. Unfortunately, cases of mineralisation were described. The cross-linking process changed to isocyanate (Pelvicol™ implant and DermMatrix™) which did not to result in calcification. Porcine small intestine submucosa has also recently been introduced(STRATASIS®).

Bovine purified pericardium is available as treated with glutaraldehyde cross-linked (UroPatch™, JAMA, Inc) or as not cross-linked, propylene oxide-treated, acellular collagen matrix (Marketed as Veritas™ Collagen Matrix).

Only small studies (level of evidence, 3–4) and one randomised trial that compared Pelvicol against TVT (Arunkalaivanan *et al.* 2003; same series followed-up by Abdel-Fattah *et al.* 2004) suggest good results at medium-term follow-up for xenografts implants that are described as biological, biocompatible, not-allergenic and rapidly incorporated into host tissue (Table 11.6). However, long-term follow-up studies are required to provide evidence of their safety and efficacy.

Table 11.5 Summary of the studies on allograft fascia lata slings for the treatment of urodynamic stress incontinence in women: main criteria

Authors	Preparation	Length of sling (cm)	Number of Patients	Follow-up months	% Cure rate of SUI	Cure rate criteria	Per cent persistent DO	Per cent de novo DO	Per cent voiding dysfunction symptoms
Wright et al. (1998)	Freeze-dried	1315	59	9.6 (1–28)	98	Clinical score	45	10	1 persistent retention (urethrolysis)
*Fitzgerald et al. (1999)	Freeze-dried irradiation	3–10	35 (32 reviewed)	3	69	Customary	Failure rate: #25% re-operation 20% autolysis of the fascia		—
Amundsen et al. (2000)	Freeze-dried	15	91	19.4 (3–37)	OCR = 63 SCR = 83	Pad used Symptoms	41	15	1 persistent retention (urethrolysis)
Elliott & Boone (2000)	Solvent-dehydrated	12	26	15 (12–20)	OCR = 77 SCR = 96	Pad used Symptoms	82	13	—
Brown & Govier (2000)	Fresh-frozen	24	104	12	74	Questionnaire	—	—	2 persistent retention
Flynn & Yap (2002)	Freeze-dried	12	63	29 (24–36)	87	Questionnaire	21	28	2 persistent retention
Chung et al. (2002)	Dermal allograft processed	3–7	19	28± 4	89	Pad used	73	5	—
Walsh et al. (2002)	Freeze-dried	10	31	12	69 85	Voiding diary Questionnaire	6	—	**3 CICS 77 obstructive symptoms
*Fitzgerald et al. (2004)	Freeze-dried irradiated	3–10	27	12 (0.5–51)	48	Telephone interview	—	—	-

*Long-term follow-up of the same series; **CICS, permanent intermittent self catheterisation; #, re-operations of eight slings' failure occurred from 5 to 9 months after surgery, DO, detrusor overactivity

In summary, autologous slings can be recommended as an effective treatment for SUI. Allograft slings provide some obvious advantages, but long-term results are not available. Xenograft slings can only be recommended for use in trials after obtaining informed consent.

Tension-free vaginal tape

The tension-free vaginal tape (TVT) procedure was introduced into clinical practice in 1994 by Petros and Ulmsten (1995) based on the new 'integral theory' concerning the mechanism of incontinence, according to which, the weakness or absence of support by the pubourethral ligaments in the middle urethra is one of the primary causes of SUI (Petros & Ulmsten 1990). The procedure is thought to work by providing mid-urethral support through a piece of prolene tape placed underneath the urethra without elevation. There are studies that try to correlate the position of the tape with the outcome, but none prove the importance of the mid-urethral position. Using a postoperative translabial ultrasound and questionnaire evaluation, Dietz *et al*. (2004) found no association between tape placement and patients' satisfaction or subjective cure rate (level 2). However, there were weak associations between more proximal tape position at Valsalva and urge incontinence ($p = 0.03$), frequency ($p = 0.048$) and symptoms of voiding dysfunction ($p = 0.029$).

The TVT appears to produce similar cure rates to the colposuspension. Four randomised controlled trials comparing TVT and Burch colposuspension (Liapis *et al*. 2002; Ward & Hilton 2004; Ward & Hilton 2002; Wang & Chen 2003) have been published (Table 11.7). Ward & Hilton (2004) described how the cure rate in their study depends on the assumptions made on the withdrawal rate. In the case of TVT, with the assumption that all dropouts were cured, the objective cure rate was 85% at two years follow-up but, with the assumption that they were failures, the objective cure rate was 63%. The operation time, hospital stay and the time to return to normal activity were significantly shorter for TVT when studied ($p < 0.001$, Ward *et al*. 2002; $p < 0.05$, Liapis 2002). Ward *et al*. (2004) found that significantly more patients in the Burch group had clinical evidence of vault or cervical prolapse and enterocoele ($p < 0.001$) and underwent surgery for pelvic organ prolapse ($p = 0.0042$), following the procedure. The authors also described a significant difference in voiding disorder requiring intermittent self-catheterisation associated with colposuspension ($p = 0.0045$). Wang *et al*. (2003) studied the effect of TVT and colposuspension on urethral obstruction using the Blaivas-Groutz nomogram and found that the difference between pre and postoperative distribution of the Burch group was significantly different ($p = 0.023$). Complications described in the four trials for the TVT procedure are reported in Table 11.7 and included bladder perforation, vaginal perforation, pelvic haematoma, tape erosion and recurrent urinary tract infections.

Two randomised trials compared TVT with laparoscopic Burch colposuspension (Paraiso *et al*. 2004; Ustun *et al*; 2003; Table 11.7) and one (Valpas *et al*. 2004) with

Table 11.6 Summary of the studies on Xenograft slings for the treatment of urodynamic stress incontinence in women. Main criteria

Authors	Type of study	Material	Length of the sling (cm)	Number of patients	Follow-up length months	Per cent cure rate	Per cent complications	Per cent postoperative voiding dysfunctions
Arunkalaivanan & Barrington (2003)	Randomised trial	Porcine dermis	10–12	A = 74 Pelvicol B = 68 TVT	12 (6–24)	A = 89 B = 85	De novo DO A = 6 B = 9	Retention: >6 weeks: A = 8.1 >1 week: B = 13.2 Sling's release: A = 7 B = 3 *CISC: A = 1 B = 4
Iosif (1987)	Prospective study	Porcine dermis	30	53	18–48	88.7	—	Retention: >2m:8
Jarvis & Fowlie (1985)	Prospective study	Porcine dermis	—	50	21 (6–48)	78	50 abdominal wound infection 2 bladder injury 14 de novo DO	—
Pelosi II et al. (2002)	Prospective study	Bovine pericardium	9	22	22 (9–26)	95	—	—

*CICS, permanent intermittent self catheterisation; w, week.

Table 11.7 Summary of randomised controlled trials, evidence level 1-2, on tension-free vaginal tape (TVT) versus other procedures for the treatment of SUI in women

Author	Procedure Voiding	Number of patients	Follow-up mean length:	Per cent OBJ cure rate	Per cent SUBJ cure rate	OBJ cure rate criteria	SUBJ cure rate criteria	Per cent De novo DO	Per cent Dysfunction Symptoms	Per cent TVT Complications
§§Ward (2004)	TVT Burch	175 169	24	63 51	25 (A) 20 (A) 43 (B) 37 (B)	1h pad-tests≤1gr	BFLUTS questionnaire: A=No leakage B=Patient's report of "cure"		Division of TVT: 1 Urethral dilation:1	see Ward 2002 + Symptoms of recurrent UTI: 5.9
§§Ward (2002)	TVT Burch	175 169	6	66 57	36 (A) 28 (A) 59 (B) 53 (B)	1h pad-tests≤1gr + cystometry	BFLUTS questionnaire: A=No leakage B=Patient's report of "cure"	TVT 8 (159 §UDS reviewed)	#CICS= TVT 3	Bladder injury: 9 Vaginal perforation: 3 Wound infection: 2 Retropubic haematoma: 2 Vascular injury: 1 Tape erosion: 1
Wang & Chen (2003)	TVT Burch	49 41	22 (12–36)	82 76	92 93	1h pad-tests≤2gr	No loss urine during exercise	Blaivas obstruction nomogram used: Pre- and post-op distribution: Burch =significantly different (p=0.0023) TVT= not significantly different (p=1.00)		—
Liapis et al. (2002)	TVT Burch	36 35	24	84 86	—	1h pad-tests≤1gr	—	16 14		Bladder perforation: 11
Paraiso et al. (2004)	TVT LBC	36 (33f-up) 36 (33 f-up)	21 (12–43)	97 81		Urodynamic evaluation	No leakage	19.3 6.2	MaxFlow rate<10 ml/sec + post-void residual volume>100: 14.7 Mesh transection: 5	Blood transfusion: 3 Bladder perforation: 6 Haematoma: 3 Pelvic abscess: 3 Mesh erosion: 2

§ UDS, urodynamics; # CICS, intermittent self catheterisation. §§. same sample of patients evaluated at different length follow-up; m, months

Table 11.7 Continued

Author	Procedure Voiding	Number of patients	Follow-up mean length:	Per cent OBJ cure rate	Per cent SUBJ cure rate	OBJ cure rate criteria	SUBJ cure rate criteria	Per cent De novo DO	Per cent Dysfunction Symptoms	Per cent TVT Complications
Valpas et al. (2004)	TVT LMC	70 51	12	85.7 56.9	82.9 58.8	Negative stress test	Subjects' expectations	urge symptom TVT = 2	Retention: 2	Bladder perforation:1 Urinary infection: 4 Wound infection 1 Bladder laceration: 8.6
Ustun et al. (2003)	TVT LBC	23 23	TVT=11 LCP=14 (3–24)	83 83		Negative stress test	No leakage	4.3	Transient urinary retention: 8.6	Bladder laceration: 8.6
§§Arunkalaivanan & Barrington (2003)	TVT Pelvicol	68 74	*12 (6–24)	A: 85 89 B: 74 76			A="dry" on symptom B= quality of life improvement> 90% + negative cough stress test	9 6	Retention: 8.3 Sling's release: TVT=3 #CISC >6w: 5 Release of sling: 2.9 Urethral dilation: 1.5	Hemorrhage >200ml: 2.9 Infection: 1.5
§§Abdel-Fattah et al. (2004)	TVT Pelvicol	68 (60 f-up) 74 (68 f-up)	*36 (12–36)		A: 79.1 77.8		Postal questionnaire: "dry" on symptom and/or quality of life improvement > 90%	15 17.6	—	—
deTayrac et al. (2004)	TVT TOT	31 (29 f-up) 30 (27 f-up)	12	83.4 90	96.8 86.7	Supine cough stress test	Subjective "satisfied" or "very satisfied"	6.7 6.5	22.6	Bladder perforation: 9.7 Urethral erosion : TVT 3.2 Urinary infection: 12.9
Rechberger et al. (2003)	TVT IVS	50 50	*13.5 (4–18)	88 80		Negative cough stress test (supine & standing position) + No leakage		16 8	Urinary retention: TVT 20	Bladder perforation: 4 Massive bleeding from bladder neck venous plexus: 4 Abdominal haematoma: 2
**Meschia et al. (2003)	TVT Fascia plication (treatment of occult stress incontinence)	25 25	*TVT = 26 *FP = 24	92 56	96 64	Cough stress test (supine position)	No symptoms of stress		Delayed voiding: TVT = 8	Bladder perforation: 4 Retropubic haematoma: 4

LBC, laparoscopic Burch colposuspension; LMC, laparoscopic mesh colposuspension; *, median value; # CICS, intermittent self catheterisation; §§, same sample of patients evaluated at different length follow-up; **, treatment of occult SUI in women with genital prolapse.

laparoscopic mesh colposuspension. They showed similar or lower cure rates with the laparoscopic procedure in the range of 83–97% for TVT and 57–83% for laparoscopic colposuspension. Operative time has been found to be significantly shorter for TVT in all trials, but there was no agreement on the length of hospital stay and catheterisation time, which were reported to be significantly longer for laparoscopic colposuspension by Ustun *et al.* ($p = 0.003$) and Valpas *et al.* ($p < 0.001$) but similar by Paraiso *et al.* ($p = 0.003$). No significant difference was found for complications.

Arunkalaivanan and Barrington (2003) randomised 142 patients to compare TVT and Pelvicol slings and found similar success rates, incidence of postoperative voiding dysfunction symptoms and *de novo* detrusor overactivity.

De Tayrac *et al.* (2004) compared tension free vaginal tape procedure with transobturator suburethral tape, recently described by Delorme (2001), who reported 90% cure rate without complications and voiding difficulties. The rates of cure described by De Tayrac *et al.* were similar for both the procedures, 83.9% versus 90% respectively, as was the incidence of complications. Mean operating time was significantly shorter for TOT ($p < 0.001$). Cystoscopy was not performed in the TOT group. It is noteworthy that the De Tayrac study was subsequently withdrawn due to ethical concerns.

Other prospective studies reported medium-term (Ulmsten 1999; Meschia *et al.* 2001), and long-term follow-up results of four to seven years (Nilsson *et al.* 2004; Nilsson *et al.* 2001; Rezapour & Ulmsten 2001a) with cure rates ranged from 82 to 90% (level 2). Long-term follow-up of four years was also described in 34 women with recurrent SUI with a cure rate of 82% (Rezapour and Ulmsten 2001b, level 2). Rardin *et al.* (2002a) described similar cure rates in patients with recurrent versus primary SUI, 85% versus 87% respectively, in a retrospective analysis of 245 women (level 3). Rezapour and Ulmsten (2001a) reported on 80 patients with mixed incontinence confirmed by urodynamics and found that 85% were cured of both stress and urge incontinence (level 2–3).

Only one randomised trial (Table 11.7) compared tension-free vaginal tape and endopelvic fascia plication in 50 women with prolapse and occult stress incontinence (Meschia *et al.* 2004, level 1) at a mean follow-up of 26 and 24 months, respectively, and found that both the subjective and objective cure rates were higher after the TVT procedure (96% versus 64%, $p = 0.01$ and 92% versus 56%, $p < 0.01$). In a prospective study of 100 women who underwent prolapse repair and TVT for occult stress incontinence, Groutz *et al.* (2004, level 3) found that postoperatively 15% patients had asymptomatic urodynamic stress incontinence. In this study 78% patients with preoperative urge incontinence had persistent urge incontinence.

Complications have been described in several studies. The most common complications reported are bladder perforation (Groutz *et al.* 2004; Karram *et al.* 2003; Levin *et al.* 2004; Table 11.7), postoperative voiding dysfunction (Klutke *et al.* 2001; Meschia 2001; Tamussino 2001a; Wang *et al.* 2002; Table 11.7) accompanied by urethral obstruction which, in some cases, required excision, release or removal of the tape (Long *et al*. 2004; Raldin *et al*, 2002b; Tzivian *et al* 2004; level of evidence, 3). *de novo* urge incontinence postoperatively (Levin *et al*. 2004; Segal *et al*. 2004; Table 11.7) has been reported in 1–20%, 1–11% and 4–22% respectively. Other rare complications reported are retropubic haematoma (Flock *et al*. 2004; Meschia 2001), severe haemorrhage in Retzius' space (Vermouth 2001), external iliac artery laceration (Milberg 2001), obdurate nerve injury (Meschia *et al*. 2001), ilea-inguinal nerve entrapment (Gees & Diet 2002), tape erosion (Tsivian 2004; Lose & Weil 2002), "post colposuspension syndrome" (consistent suprapubic pain directly over the ileo-pectineal ligament) (Barrington *et al*. 2002; level 4), necrotising fasciitis (Johnson 2003), bowel perforation (Meschia *et al*. 2002; Tamussino 2001b) or delayed bowel erosion (Fourie & Cohen 2003).

In a randomised trial, Rechberger *et al*. (2003) compared elastic monofilament, inserted with the TVT device (Gynecare) with a less elastic multifilament polypropylene tape, inserted by the IVS (Tyco) instrument. The cure rates were similar, but there was a statistical difference in the incidence of postoperative urinary retention ($p = 0.023$), greater for the TVT. However, a case-controlled study showed a greater incidence of erosion following the IVS than the TVT (14% versus less than 1% respectively) which the authors related to the type of the mesh used (Glavin & Sander 2003, level 3).

In summary, randomised controlled trials with follow-up to two years showed similar cure rates between TVT, open and laparoscopic colposuspension (level of evidence, 1–2). When TVT has been compared with porcine slings, TOT and multifilament material, one year follow-up showed similar cure rates (level of evidence, 1–2). Long-term follow-up of seven years reported has demonstrated an objective cure rate of 81% (level of evidence, 2). One randomised trial found a significantly higher cure rate for TVT when the procedure was compared with endopelvic fascia plication for the treatment of occult SUI during prolapse repairs (level 1).

Injectable agents

Periurethral bulking agents have been used since 1938 when Murless injected a sclerosing solution into the anterior vaginal wall in 20 women, causing a fibrous reaction and subsequent continence. Since then, many bulking agents have been described. The prime indication was originally thought to be intrinsic sphincter deficiency without urethral hypermobility, but similar outcomes have been reported with hypermobility (Bent *et al*. 2001; Kholi *et al*. 2000; Monga 1995). However, there is no clear indication on which urodynamic parameter should be used to define intrinsic sphincter deficiency and on the meaning of urethral hypermobility. It appears that the therapeutic mechanism is an increase in urethral resistance, but this has not been proved. Paraurethral or transurethral methods of delivery of the bulking agents have been described under local anaesthesia, but the correct location of injection, volume of the agent, numbers of reinjection in each session and type of instrument used have not been defined. Many variations have been described. As with many papers on continence treatment, there is no consistent definition of cure, with follow-up rarely longer than one year and often with a small number of women recruited.

The bulking agent should be hypoallergenic, biocompatible and non immunogenic. It should cause minimal inflammatory and fibrotic reactions and should be permanent. The latter characteristic is determined by the particle size. They have to be greater than 80 μm to avoid macrophage phagocytosis and migration. Particle absorption is thought to contribute to eventual failure or recurrence (Chrouser *et al.* 2004).

GAX-collagen (glutaraldehyde-cross-linked bovine collagen, Contigen) has been one of the most frequently used injectable agents. It may cause allergic reactions (Leonard *et al.* 1990) and requires a skin-test. Autologous fat avoids hypersensitivity related to foreign materials, but has been related to rapid digestion and potential migration (Lightner 2002). Carbon beads, Durasphere, with diameter of 250–300 μm, are designed to avoid migration (Lightner *et al.* 2001; Carvosa *et al.* 2000). However, Pannek *et al.* (2001) has described carbon beads migration in local and distant lymph nodes in two patients three months after the injection. Silicone particles, Macroplastique, have been used since 1991 and consist of particles >100 μm that avoid migration (Henalla *et al.* 2000). Polytetrafluoroethylene particles (Teflon) are sized between 4 and 40 μm and have shown migration with granuloma formations and emboli in lung, liver, lymph nodes, kidneys, spleen and brain (Malizia *et al.*1984; Mittleman & Maraccini 1983) which led to its withdrawal. Other materials recently introduced are calcium idroxylapatite, coaptite (Dmochowsky 2002), and ethylene vinyl alcohol copolymer, EVOH, (Dmochowsky 2002b).

Pikard *et al.* (2004) recently reviewed seven randomised or quasi randomised trials in which one management arm included bulking agents. Only one trial compared placebo with autologous fat, but it was interrupted early for safety reasons. Three month follow-up was reported and showed similar results (Lee *et al.* 2001). One study compared injectable agents with different open surgical procedures (Corcos *et al.* 2001) and with a year follow-up found that the subjective cure rates were similar but there was a statistically significant difference in objective cure rate, evaluated with 24 hours pad-test, favouring the open procedure (cure rates 53% versus 72%; RR 1.69; 95% CI 1.02–2.79). Complications and their severity were significantly higher in the surgical procedure group. Two studies compared different agents and found that silicone particles and carbon beads showed the same outcome as collagen at one year follow-up (Anders 1999; Lightner 2001). Dmokowski (2002a, b) compared new agents such as coaptite and uryx with collagen, but only subjective outcomes were described and they were similar in each group. Finally, Nager (1998) compared paraurethral and transurethral injection and described similar outcomes at one month evaluation but found a higher incidence of retention in the first arm (30% versus 5% respectively).

Most studies reported are case series (level 4 evidence) with heterogeneous populations and different cure rate criteria (Table 11.8). The average cure rate for GAX-collagen ranges from 7 to 44% in the literature. The most frequent post-procedure complications have been *de novo* urgency with an incidence up to 12.6%, haematuria in 5% of cases (Stothers *et al.* 1998), urinary retention and urinary infections ranging from 1% to 8% and from 0.5% to 4% respectively (Hershorn *et al.* 1995; Winters & Appell 1995). The objective cure rate for Carbon beads has been reported from 33% to 61% at 9–12 month follow-up (Lightner *et al.* 2001; Pannek *et al.* 2001; Table 11.8) but again, data were not clearly expressed. Particle migration, an important complication, has been reported with Durasphere, (Pannek *et al.* 2000). Autologous fat material has been used and has the obvious attraction of being cheap and readily available. The average cure rate reported in several case series studies has been 13–50% (Su *et al.* 1998; Trokman *et al.* 1995; see Table 11.8) with a time-dependent decrease in efficacy (Santarosa *et al.* 1994), but the only randomised trial available (Lee *et al.* 2002) found no difference in the outcome when autologous fat was compared with placebo. Complications such as infections and urinary retention have been reported with fat and, unfortunately, cases of death due to lung embolism have been described (Currie *et al.* 1997; Lee *et al.* 2001). Since 1991, Macroplastique has been used for both intrinsic sphincter deficiency and urethral hypermobility and the cure rates reported were 14–67% and 0–20%, respectively (Table 11.8). Koelbl *et al.* (1998), and Usman and Henalla (1998) described a time-dependent decrease in efficacy. Few complications such as *de novo* urgency, urinary infections, haematuria and urinary retention were found, but no serious complications or migration of the particles.

In general, urethral injection with bulking agents represents a minimally invasive procedure for SUI which may be performed in the outpatient setting. Although short term follow-up showed good cure rates (level 4 evidence), a time-dependent decrease in efficacy has been observed. It is still unclear whether some of the new agents available offer better medium and long-term results than the 20% improvement rate seen with collagen at five years follow-up. There is no evidence to prove that one agent is better than another (level of evidence, 4).

Although injectable agents may be recommended as a low risk form of treatment for stress incontinence, the patient must be counselled about the low cure rate and the small risk of irritative and voiding symptoms after treatment.

Further long-term clinical randomised trials using objective measures of outcome are needed to establish the long-term efficacy and safety of different bulking agents.

Table 11.8 Summary of studies of bulking agents approved by FDA: autologous fat, carbon beads (Durasphere), GAX collagen, and macroplastique for periurethral injection for the treatment of SUI in women

Authors	Type of study	Number of injections	Volume of injected agent	Number of patients	Follow-up mean length (months)	% Cure rate and improvement	Level of evidence
Summary of autologous fat series							
Lee et al. (2001)	RCT (fat injection/ placebo, saline)	2–3 (fat) 3 (placebo)	—	35 fat, A- (27 f-up) 33 saline,B (26 f-up)	3	OBJ + SUBJ A: cured 22.2 B: cured 20.7	1–2
Su et al. (1998)	Case series	1	14.8 ml	26	17.4	OBJ: cured 50 improved15.4	4
Haab et al. (1997b)§§NRPCT (fat injection / collagen)		1.6	12.1 ml	45 fat, A 22 collagen, B	7	SUBJ: Cured:A 13; B 24 Improved: A 32; B 71	2–3
Trockman et al. (1995)	Case series	1.6	21.3 ml	32	6	SUBJ: Cured 13 Improved 44	4
Blaivas et al. (1994)	Case series	2.7	12 ml (5–25)	45	12	OBJ + SUBJ Cured 28 Improved 51	4
Santarosa & Blaivas (1994)	Case series	2.4 (1–4)	5–15 ml	12	18 (12–30)	OBJ + SUBJ Cured 57	4
Summary of carbon beads (Durasphere) series							
Chrouser et al. (2004)	Retrospective comparative series (A)Durasphere/ (B)GAXcollagen	Not mentioned	Not mentioned	56 (43 follow-up)	*51(A) *62 (B)	SUBJ (A) 21 (B) 5	2
Madjar et al. (2003)	Case series	Same position of the needle (4 o'clock)	1 ml/2–3	70 (46 f-up)	9.4 (3–18)	SUBJ cured 52.2 improved 13	4
Lightner et al. (2001)	RCT (collagen versus carbon beads)	Same position of the needle (4 o'clock)	4.83 ml	178	12	OBJ: Cured 61	1
Pannek et al. (2001)	Case series	3	6 cm³ (3–9)	20	12	OBJ: Cured 33	4

RCT, randomised controlled trial; §§, non-randomised comparative prospective study: autologous fat versus collagen; *, median length of follow-up.

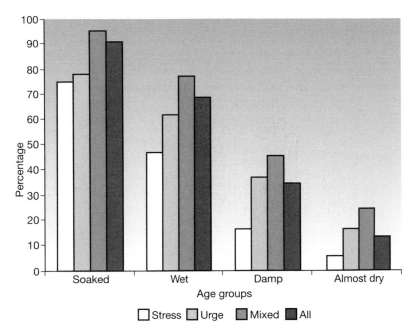

Figure 4.4 Bothersome incontinence by severity in women

confounded by increasing severity in older age. To identify factors that are independently associated with quality of life impairment, a multivariate logistic regression analysis was carried out. Age, severity and type of incontinence were entered into the model (see Table 4.1). Both severity and type of incontinence independently predicted social disability and bothersomeness. Women who were soaked or wet were more likely to experience impaired quality of life compared to those who had minimal leakage (almost dry). The variation in impact of the different types of incontinence was borne out in the multivariate analysis, with women having urge and mixed symptoms being more likely than those with stress symptoms to have quality of life impairments.

However, only the oldest age groups were more likely to be bothered by symptoms, but not disabled, than the youngest group of 40–49 year olds. This analysis supports the contention that some of the age effects are confounded by severity and type of incontinence.

Relationship between social disability and help-seeking

Although the data presented show SUI to be a very common symptom in women, relatively few seek help from a healthcare professional. Estimates of help-seeking range from around 9% (Samuelsson *et al.* 1997) to as many as 88% (Brown *et al.*

Table 11.8 Continued

Summary of collagen series

Authors	Type of study	Number of injections	Volume of injected agent (ml) (mean)	Number of patients	Follow-up mean length (months)	Per cent cure rate (cure and improvement)	Level of evidence
Bent et al. (2001)	Multi-centre prospective study	1–3	#13.4 (2.5–37.5)	Total 90 (A) ISD+ HU 58 (B)	12	SUBJ (A) cured 21 improved 21 (B)cured 33 improved 33	4
Gorton et al. (1999)	Retrospective study	2–3	^17 (4–65)	61 (37> 60months f-up)	24 >60	OBJ: cured 18 SUBJ: improved 35 SUBJ (questionnaire) Cured: no pad used 3 Improved 35	4
Corcos & Furnier (1999)	Case series	2.2	9	40	50	cured 30 improved 40	4
Elsergany et al. (1998)5	Case series	—	6.1 (previous 11) 3.5 (last 22)	33	18.8	OBJ cured 48 improved 33.3	4
Smith et al. (1997)	Case series	2	11.9	35	12	SUBJ: Cured + improved 83	4
Swami et al. (1997)	Case series	—	—	111	39	SUBJ cured 25 improved 40	4
Monga et al. (1995)	Case series	1.6	11.7	60	24	OBJ: Cured 48	4
O'Connell et al. (1995)	Case series	1.5	9.1	44		SUBJ: Cured 63	4
Winters et al. (1995)	Case series	—	—	160	24	SUBJ: Cured+ improved 78	4
Herschorn et al. (1992)	Case series	2	12.7	31	6	OBJ: Cured 48 Improved 42	4

#, cumulative volume injected; IDS, intrinsic sphincter deficiency; ^, median value.

Table 11.8 Continued

Summary of macroplastique series

Authors	Type of study	Number of injections	Volume of injected agent	Number of patients	Follow-up mean length (months)	Per cent cure rate	Level of evidence
Tamanini et al. (2003)	Case series	3 (1 session)	6.3 ml	21	12	62 (pad test) 40 UDS 57.1 SUBJ	4
°°Gurdal et al. (2002)	Comparative prospective study	1	3.5 ml	15 ISD (A) 14 ISD + HM (B)	24	SUBJ: cured 66.7 (A); 21.4 (B) improved 13.3 (A); 13.3 (B)	4
Radley et al. (2001)	Case series	1.47	6.73 ml	56ISD 41ISD + HU	19 SUBJ 16 OBJ	SUBJ: Cured 19.6; improved 39.3 OBJ: Cured 39 4	4
Barranger et al. (2000)	Case series	1	4 ml	21 ISD (A) 6 ISD + HU (B)	31 (24–34)	SUBJ: (A) = Cured 19; improved 29 (B) = Cured and improved 0	4
Henalla et al. (2000)	Multicentre prospective study	3 (_two sessions)	5 ml	40 (39 follow-up)	3	SUBJ:41 cured 33.3 improved	4
Koelbl et al. (1998)	Case series	1.13	3.9 ml	32 ISD	6 12	SUBJ+ OBJ: Cured 75 Cured 59	4
Usman & Henalla (1998)	Retrospective comparative study	1	5 ml	71ISD (P) 31 ISD (S)	3 [all patients] 17.6 (11–44) [P=58 patients S=28 patients]	SUBJ: P = Cured 30; improved 37 S = Cured 42; improved 29 SUBJ: P = Cured 23; improved 25 S = Cured 14; improved 32 3	4
Sheriff et al. (1997)	Case series	1.19	5 ml	(A) 34 ISD (B) 7 ISD+HU (C) 2 NS	24 (A) 3 (B + C)	SUBJ: A = failure rate 52 (B°C) = failure rate 100	4
°°Harriss et al. (1996)	Case series	1.25	2–7 ml	40 ISD	36 SUBJ 3 OBJ + SUBJ	SUBJ: Cured 40; improved 18 OBJ +SUBJ: Cured 40; improved 33	4

IDS, intrinsic sphincter deficiency; HU, urethral hypermobility; NS, neuropathic sphincter; P, primary treatment; S, secondary treatment; previous failed incontinence surgery °°, periurethral injection.

Conclusions

The evidence for any surgical procedure for the treatment of SUI is often limited by the poor quality of studies, small size of samples and different outcome measurements used. Only a few randomised trials have been published and even fewer have the power to determine the value of the procedures studied. Outcome measures employed, even when objective, often correlate poorly with patients' perception of their treatment. Peri-operative complications, postoperative pain and long-term complications such as voiding dysfunction, detrusor overactivity and prolapse must be reported. Economic outcomes should be studied in the comparison of different procedures for a complete evaluation.

References

Abdel-Fattah, M. *et al.* (2004). Pelvicol™ pubovaginal sling versus Tension-Free Vaginal Tape for treatment of urodynamic stress incontinence: a prospective randomised three year follow-up study. *European Urology* **46**, 629–635.

Abrams, P. *et al.* (2002). Second International Consultation on Incontinence, Recommendations of the International Scientific Committee: Evaluation and Treatment of Urinary Incontinence, Pelvic Organ Prolapse and Faecal Incontinence, Paris 1–3 2001

Alcalay, M. *et al.* (1995). Burch colposuspension: a 10–20 year follow up. *British Journal of Obstetrics and Gynecology* **102**, 740–745.

Amundsen, C. L. *et al.* (2000). Outcome in 104 pubovaginal slings using freeze-dried allograft from a single tissue bank. *Urology* **56** (Suppl. 6A), 2–8.

Anders, K. *et al.* (1999). Gax collagen or macroplastique does it make a difference? [abstract]. *International Urogynecology Journal and Pelvic Floor Dysfunction* **10** (Suppl. 1), S46.

Ankardal, M. (2004). A randomised trial comparing open Burch colposuspension using sutures with laparoscopic colposuspension using mesh and staples in women with stress urinary incontinence. *British Journal of Obstetrics and Gynecology* **111**, 974–981.

Arunkalaivanan, A. S. & Barrington, J. W. (2003). Randomised trial of porcine dermal sling (Pelvicol™ implant) vs tension free vaginal tape (TVT) in the surgical treatment of stress incontinence: a questionnaire based study. *International Urogynecology Journal and Pelvic Floor Dysfunction* **14**, 17–23.

Aslan, P. & Woo, H. H. (1997). Ureteric injury following laparoscopic colposuspension. *British Journal of Obstetrics and Gynaecology* **104**, 266–268.

Barranger, E. *et al.* (2000). Results of transurethral injection of silicone micro-implants for women with intrinsic sphincter deficiency. *Journal of Urology* **164**, 1619–1622.

Barrington, J. W. *et al.* (2002). Post-colposuspension syndrome following a Tension-Free Vaginal Tape procedure. *International Urogynecology Journal and Pelvic Floor Dysfunction*, **13**, 187–188.

Barrington, J. W. *et al.* (1998). The modified rectus fascial sling for the treatment of genuine stress incontinence. *Journal of Obstetrics and Gynecology* **18**, 61–62.

Beck, R. P. *et al.* (1991). A 25-years experience with 519 anterior colporrhaphy procedures. *Obstetrics and Gynecology* **78**, 1011–1018.

Beck, R. P. *et al.* (1988). The fascia lata sling procedure for treating recurrent genuine stress incontinence of urine. *Obstetrics and Gynecology* **72**, 699–703.

Bent, A. *et al.* (2001). Collagen Implant for treating stress urinary incontinence in women with urethral hypermobility. *Journal of Urology* **166**, 1354–1357.

Bergman, A. & Elia, G. (1995). Three surgical procedures for genuine stress incontinence: Five-year follow-up of a prospective randomized study. *American Journal of Obstetrics and Gynaecology* **173**, 66–71.

Bergman, A. *et al.* (1989). Comparison of three different surgical procedures for genuine stress incontinence. Prospective randomised study. *American Journal of Obstetrics and Gynaecology* **161**, 1102–1106.

Black, N. A. & Downs, S. H. (1996). The effectiveness of surgery for stress incontinence in women: a systematic review. *British Journal of Urology* **78**, 497–510.

Blaivas, J. G. *et al.* (1994). Periurethral fat injection for sphincteric incontinence in women. *Journal of Urology* **151**, 419A.

Bombieri, L. *et al.* (2002a). Objective assessment of bladder neck elevation and urethral compression at colposuspension. *British Journal of Obstetrics and Gynaecology* **109**, 395–401.

Bombieri, L. *et al.* (2002b). Why do women have voiding dysfunction and de novo detrusor instability after colposuspension? *British Journal of Obstetrics and Gynaecology* **109**, 402–412.

Breen, J. M. *et al.* (1997). The fascia lata suburethral sling for treating recurrent urinary stress incontinence. *American Journal of Obstetrics and Gynaecology* **177**, 1363–1275.

Brown, S. L. & Govier, F. E. (2000). Cadaveric versus autologous fascia lata for the pubovaginal sling: surgical outcome and patient satisfaction. *Journal of Urology* **164**, 1633–1637.

Burch, J. C. (1968). Cooper's ligaments urethrovesical suspension for stress incontinence. Nine years' experience, results, complications, technique. *American Journal of Obstetrics and Gynecology* **100**, 764–774.

Burton, G. (1997). A three year prospective randomised urodynamic study comparing open and laparoscopic colposuspension. *Neurourology and Urodynamics* **16**, 353–354.

Carey, M. *et al.* (2000). Laparoscopic versus open colposuspension: a prospective multicentre randomised single-blind comparison. *Neurourology and Urodynamics* **19**, 389–391.

Chaikin, D. C. *et al.* (1998). Pubovaginal fascia sling for all type of stress urinary incontinence: long term analysis. *Journal of Urology* **160**, 1312–1316.

Chou, E. C. L. *et al.* (2003). Effective treatment for mixed urinary incontinence with a pubovaginal sling. *Journal of Urology* **170**, 494–497.

Chung, S. J. *et al.* (2002). Technique of combined pubovaginal sling and cystocoele repair using a single piece of cadaveric dermal graft. *Urology* **59**, 538–541.

Clemens, J. Q. *et al.* (1998). Long term results of the Stamey bladder neck suspension: direct comparison with the Marshall-Marchetti-Krantz procedure. *Journal of Urology* **160**, 372–376.

Colombo, M. *et al.* (2000). Randomised comparison of Burch colposuspension versus anterior colporrhaphy in women with stress urinary incontinence and anterior vaginal wall prolapse. *British Journal of Obstetrics and Gynaecology* **107**, 544–551.

Colombo, M. *et al.* (1996). A randomised comparison of Burch colposuspension and anterior paravaginal defect for female stress urinary incontinence. *American Journal of Obstetrics and Gynecology* **175**, 78–84.

Colombo, M. *et al.* (1994). Burch colposuspension versus modified versus modified Marshall-Marchetti-Krantz urethropexy for primary genuine stress incontinence: a prospective randomised clinical trial. *American Journal of Obstetrics and Gynecology* **171**, 1573–1579.

Cooper, J. L. & Beck, C. L. (1993). History of soft tissue allografts in orthopaedics. *Sports Medicine and Arthroscopy Review* **1**, 2–16.

Corcos, J. *et al.* (2001). Surgery versus collagen for the treatment of female stress urinary incontinence (SUI): 1 year follow-up results of a multicentre randomised trial (RCT)[abstract]. Proceedings of the International Continence Society (ICS), 31st Annual Meeting, Seoul, Korea, 18–21 September 2001: abstract 248.

Corcos, J. & Fournier, C. (1999). Periurethral collagen injection for the treatment of female stress urinary incontinence: 4 year follow-up results. *Urology* **54**, 815–818.

Costantini, E. *et al.* (2003). Four-corner colposuspension: clinical and functional results. *International Urogynecology Journal of Pelvic Floor Dysfunction* **14**, 113–118.

Cross, C. A. *et al.* (1998). Our experience with pubovaginal slings in patients with Stress Urinary Incontinence. *Journal of Urology* **159**, 1195–1198.

Culligan, J. *et al.* (2003). A randomized controlled trial comparing a modified Burch procedure and suburethral sling: long-term follow-up. *International Urogynecology Journal and Pelvic Floor Dysfunction* **14**, 229–233.

Currie, I. *et al.* (1997). Adipose tissue and lipid droplet embolism following periurethral injection of autologous fat: case report and review of the literature. *International Urogynecology Journal and Pelvic Floor Dysfunction* **8**, 377–380.

Czapliki, M. *et al.* (1998). Long Term Subjective results of Marshall-Marchetti-Krantz procedure. *European Urology* **34**, 118–123.

Delorme, E. (2001). Transobturator urethral suspension: mini-invasive procedure in the treatment of stress urinary incontinence in women. *Progress in Urology* **11**, 1306–1313.

deTayrac, R. *et al.* (2004). A prospective randomised trial comparing tension-free vaginal tape and transobturator suburethral tape for the treatment of stress urinary incontinence. *American Journal of Obstetrics and Gynecology* **190**, 602–608.

Dolan, L. *et al.* (2004). Opening Detrusor Pressure and Influence of Age on Success Following Colposuspension. *Neurourology and Urodynamics* **23**, 10–15.

Dmochowski, R. *et al.* (2002a). Initial clinical results from coaptite injection for stress urinary incontinence comparative clinical study [abstract]. Proceedings of the International Continence Society (ICS), 32nd Annual Meeting, Heidelberg, Germany 28–30 August 2002, pp. 184–185.

Dmochowski, R. *et al.* (2002b). Multicentre randomized controlled study to evaluate uryx urethral bulking agent in treating female stress urinary incontinence [abstract]. Proceedings of the International Continence Society (ICS), 32nd Annual Meeting, Heidelberg, Germany 28–30 August 2002, p. 187.

Digesu, G. A. *et al.* (2004). Effects of Burch colposuspension on the relative positions of the bladder neck to the elevator ani muscle: An observational study that used magnetic resonance imaging. *American Journal of Obstetrics and Gynecology* **190**, 164–169.

Dietz, H. P. *et al.* (2004). How important is TVT location? *Acta Obstetricia et Gynecologica Scandinavica* **83**, 904–908.

Dwyen, P.L. *et al.* (1999). Suture injury to the urinary tract in urethral suspension procedures for stress incontinence. *International Urogynecology Journal and Pelvic Floor Dysfunction* **10**, 15–21.

Elliott, D. S. & Boone, T. B. (2000). Is fascia lata allografts material trustworthy for pubovaginal sling repair? *The Journal of Urology* **56**, 772–776.

Elsergany, R. *et al.* (1998). Transurethral collagen injection for female stress incontinence. *International Urogynecology Journal and Pelvic Floor Dysfunction* **9**, 13–18.

Enzelsberger, H. *et al.* (1996). Comparison of Burch and Lyodura sling procedures for repair of unsuccessful incontinence surgery. *Obstetrics & Gynecology* **88**, 251–256.

Fatty, H. *et al.* (2001). Modified Burch colposuspension: Laparoscopy versus Laparotomy. *Journal of the American Association of Gynecologic Laparoscopists* **8**, 99–106.

Fitzgerald, M. P. *et al.* (2004). Medium-term follow-up on use of freeze-dried, irradiated donor fascia for sacrocolpopexy and sling procedures. *International Urogynecology Journal and Pelvic Floor Dysfunction* **15**, 233–242.

Fitzgerald, M. P. *et al.* (1999). Failure of allograft suburethral slings. *British Journal of Urology* **84**, 785–788.

Flock, F. *et al.* (2004). Hemorrhagic complications associated with tension free vaginal tape procedure. *Obstetrics and Gynecology* **104**, 989–994.

Flynn, B. & Yap, W. T. (2002). Pubovaginal sling using allogaft fascia lata versus autograft fascia lata for all types of stress urinary incontinence: 2 years minimum follow-up. *Journal of Urology* **167**, 608–612.

Fourie, T. & Cohen, P. L. (2003). Delayed bowel erosion by tension-free vaginal tape. *International Urogynecology Journal and Pelvic Floor Dysfunction* **14**, 362–364.

Geis, K. & Dietl, J. (2002). Ileo-inguinal nerve entrapment after Tension-Free Vaginal Tape procedure. *International Urogynecology Journal and Pelvic Floor Dysfunction* **13**, 136–138.

Gittes, R. F. & Loughlin, K. R. (1987). No-incision pubo-vaginal suspension for stress incontinence. *Journal of Urology* **138**, 568–570.

Gilja, I. (2000). Transvaginal needle suspension operation: the way we do it. Clinical and urodynamic study: long-term results. *European Urology* **37**, 325–330.

Glavin, K. & Sander, P. (2004). Erosion, defecting healing and extrusion after tension free urethropexy for the treatment of stress urinary incontinence. *International Urogynecology Journal and Pelvic Floor Dysfunction* **15**, 179–182.

Glazener, C. M. A. & Cooper, K. (2004). Anterior vaginal repair for urinary incontinence in women (Cochrane Review). In *The Cochrane Library*, issue 3.

Glazener, C. M. A. & Cooper, K. (2004). Bladder neck needle suspension for urinary incontinence in women (Cochrane Review). In *The Cochrane Library*, issue 3.

Golomb, J. *et al.* (1997). Suspended pubovaginal fascial sling for the correction of complicated stress urinary incontinence. *European Urology* **32**, 170–174.

Golomb, J. *et al.* (2001). Management of urethral erosion caused by a pubovaginal fascia sling. *Urology* **57**, 159–160.

Gorton, E. *et al.* (1999). Periurethral collagen injection: a long-term follow-up study. *British Journal of Urology* **84**, 966–971.

Govier, F. E. *et al.* (1997). Pubovaginal slings using fascia lata for the treatment of intrinsic sphincter deficiency. *Journal of Urology* **157**, 117–121.

Grountz, A. *et al.* (2004). Tension-Free Vaginal Tape (TVT) for the treatment of occult stress urinary incontinence in women undergoing prolapse repair: a prospective study of 100 consecutive cases. *Neurourology and Urodynamics* **23**, 632–635.

Grountz, A. *et al.* (2001). Pubovaginal sling surgery for simple stress urinary incontinence: analysis by an outcome score. *Journal of Urology* **165**, 1597–1560.

Gurdal, M. *et al.* (2002). Endoscopic silicone injection for female stress urinary incontinence due to sphincter deficiency: impact of coexisting urethral mobility on treatment outcome. *Journal of Urology* **60**, 1016–1019.

Haab, F. *et al.* (1997a). Results of pubovaginal sling for the treatment of intrinsic sphincteric deficiency determined by questionnaire analysis. *Journal of Urology* **158**, 1738–1741.

Haab, F. *et al.* (1997b). Urinary stress incontinence due to intrinsic sphincteric deficiency: experience with fat and collagen periurethral injection. *Journal of Urology* **157**, 1283–1286.

Handa, V. *et al.* (1996). Banked Human Fascia Lata for the Suburethral Sling Procedure: A Preliminary Report. *American Journal of Obstetrics and Gynecology* **88**, 1045–1049.

Harriss, D. R. *et al.* (1996). Periurethral silicone micro-implants (Macroplastique) for the treatment of genuine stress incontinence. *British Journal of Urology* **78**, 722–726.

Hassouna, M. E. & Ghoniem, G. M. (1999). Long-term outcome and quality of life after modified pubovaginal sling for intrinsic sphincter deficiency. *Urology* **53**, 287–291.

Hegarty, P. K. *et al.* (2001). Longevity of the Marshall-Marchetti-Krantz procedure. *Annales Chirurgiae et Gynaecologiae* **90**, 286–289.

Herschorn, S. *et al.* (1992). Early experience with intraurethral collagen injection for urinary incontinence. *Journal of Urology* **148**, 1797–1800.

Hilton, P. (2002). Trials surgery for stress incontinence-thoughts on the "Humpty Dumpty principle". *British Journal of Obstetrics and Gynaecology* **109**, 1081–1088.

Hilton, P. & Mayne, C. J. (1991). The Stamey endoscopic bladder neck suspension: a clinical and urodynamic investigation, including actuarial follow-up over four years. *British Journal of Obstetrics and Gynaecology* **98**, 1141–1149.

Hutchings, A. & Black, N. A. (2001). Surgery for stress incontinence: a non randomised trial of colposuspension, needle suspension and anterior colporrhaphy. *European Urology* **39**, 375–382.

Iosif, C. S. (1987). Porcine corium sling in the treatment of urinary stress incontinence. *Archives of Gynecology* **240**, 131–136.

Jarvis, G. J. & Foulie, A. (1985). Clinical and urodynamic assessment of the porcine dermis bladder sling in the treatment of genuine stress incontinence. *British Journal of Obstetrics and Gynaecology* **92**, 1189–1191.

Jeffrey, M. *et al.* (2000). The rectus muscle suburethral sling as a treatment for complicated stress urinary incontinence. *Obstetrics and Gynecology* **95**, S19–S20.

Johnson, D. W. *et al.* (2003). Necrotizing fasciitis after tension-free vaginal tape (TVT) placement. *International Urogynecology Journal and Pelvic Floor Dysfunction* **14**, 291–293.

Kammerer-Doak, D. *et al.* (1999). A Randomized Trial of Burch Retropubic Urethropexy and Anterior Colporrhaphy for Stress Urinary Incontinence. *Obstetrics and Gynecology* **93**, 75–78.

Kammerer-Doak, D. *et al.* (1998). Osteitis Pubis after Marshall-Marchetti-Kranz urethropexy: A pubic osteomyelitis. *American Journal of Obstetrics and Gynecology* **179**, 586–590.

Kane, L. *et al.* (1999). The pubofascial anchor sling procedure for recurrent genuine urinary stress incontinence. *British Journal of Urology* **83**, 1010–1014.

Karram, M. M. *et al.* (2003). Complications and untoward effects of the Tension-Free Vaginal Tape procedure. *Obstetrics and Gynecology* **101**, 929–932.

Kenton, K. *et al.* (2002). Multiple foreign body erosion after laparoscopic colposuspension with mesh. *American Journal of Obstetrics and Gynecology* **187**, 252–253.

Klutke, J. J. *et al.* (2000). Transvaginal Bladder Neck Suspension with Cooper's Ligaments Fixation. *Journal of Reproductive Medicine* **45**, 541–545.

Koelbl, H. *et al.* (1998). Transurethral injection of silicone micro-implants for intrinsic sphincter urethral deficiency. *Obstetrics and Gynecology* **92**, 332–336.

Kreder, K. J. & Winfield, H. N. (1997). Laparoscopic urethral sling for treatment of intrinsic sphincter deficiency. *Journal of Endourology* **10**, 255–257.

Kwon, C. *et al.* (2003). The development of pelvic organ prolapse following isolated Burch retropubic uretropexy. *International Urogynecology Journal and Pelvic Floor Dysfunction* **14**, 321–25.

Langer, R. *et al.* (2001). Long term follow up after Burch colposuspension for urinary stress incontinence. *International Urogynecology Journal and Pelvic Floor Dysfunction* **12**, 323–27.

Latini, J. M. *et al.* (2004). Efficacy and morbidity of autologous fascia sling cystourethropexy. *The Journal of Urology* **171**, 1180–1184.

Leach, G. E. *et al.* (1997). Female Stress Urinary Incontinence Clinical Guidelines Panel summary report on surgical management of female stress urinary incontinence. *Journal of Urology* **158**, 875–880.

Lee, P. (2001). Periurethral autologous fat injection as treatment for female stress urinary incontinence. A randomised, double-blind controlled trial. *Journal of Urology* **165**, 153–158.

Lemer, M. L. *et al.* (1999). Tissue strength analysis of autologous and cadaveric allografts for the pubo-vaginal sling. *Neurourology and Urodynamics* **18**, 497–453.

Leonard, M. P. *et al.* (1990). Local tissue reaction to the suburethral injection of glutaraldehyde cross-linked bovine collagen in humans. *Journal of Urology* **143**, 1209–1212.

Levin, I. *et al.* (2004). Surgical complications and medium-term outcome results of Tension-Free Vaginal Tape: a prospective study of 313 consecutive patients. *Neurourology and Urodynamics* **23**, 7–9.

Liapis, A. *et al.* (2002). Burch colposuspension and tension-free vaginal tape in the management of stress urinary incontinence in women. *European Urology* **41**, 469–473.

Liapis, A. *et al.* (1996). Genuine stress incontinence: Prospective randomized comparison two operative methods. *European Journal of Obstetrics, Gynecology and Reproductive Biology* **64**, 69–72.

Lightner, D. *et al.* (2001). A new injectable bulking agent for treatment of stress urinary incontinence: results of a multi-centre, randomised, controlled, double-blind study of Durasphere™. *Urology* **58**, 12–15.

Lohse, C. & Weil A. (2002). A rare complication with TVT: vaginal protrusion of the tape. *International Urogynecology Journal and Pelvic Floor Dysfunction* 13, 330–331.

Loughlin K. R. *et al.* (1996). The endoscopic fascial sling for treatment of female urinary stress incontinence. *Journal of Urology* **155**, 1265–1267.

Long, C. Y. L. *et al.* (2004). Lateral Excision of Tension-Free Vaginal Tape for the Treatment of Iatrogenic Urethral Obstruction. *Obstetrics and Gynaecology* **104**, 1270–1274.

Madjar S. *et al.* (2003). New periurethral bulking agents for stress urinary incontinence: modified technique and early results. *Journal of Urology* **170**, 2327–2329.

Malizia, A. *et al.* (1984). Migration and granulomatous reaction after periurethral injection of polytef (Teflon). *Journal of the American Medical Association* **251**, 3277–3281.

Maher, C. *et al.* (1999). The Burch colposuspension for recurrent urinary stress incontinence following retropubic continence surgery. *British Journal of Obstetrics and Gynaecology* **106**, 719–724.

Mainprize, T. C. & Drutz, H. P. (1988). The Marshall-Marchetti-Krantz procedure: a critical review. *Obstetrical Gynecological Survey* **43**, 724–729.

Mallipeddi, P. K. *et al.* (2001). Anatomic and functional outcome of vaginal paravaginal repair in the correction of anterior vaginal wall prolapse. *International Urogynecology Journal and Pelvic Floor Dysfunction* **12**, 83–88.

Mason, R. C. & Roach, M. (1996). Modified pubovaginal sling for treatment of intrinsic sphincteric deficiency. *Journal of Urology* **156**, 1991–1994.

Masson, D. B. & Govier, F. E. (2000). Modified Pereyra bladder neck suspension in patients with intrinsic sphincter deficiency and bladder neck hypermobility: patients' satisfaction with a mean follow-up of 4 years. *Urology* **55**, 217–221.

McLennan, M. T. *et al.* (1998). Clinical and Urodynamic Predictors of Delayed Voiding After Fascia Lata Suburethral Sling. *Obstetrics and Gynecology* **92**, 608–612.

Meschia, M. *et al.* (2003). A randomised comparison of tension-free vaginal tape and endopelvic fascia placation in women with genital prolapse and occult stress urinary incontinence. *American Journal of Obstetrics and Gynecology* **190**, 609–613.

Meschia, M. *et al.* (2002). Bowel perforation during insertion of tension-free vaginal tape. *International Urogynecology Journal and Pelvic Floor Dysfunction* **13**, 263–265.

Meschia, M. *et al.* (2001). Tension free vaginal tape: analysis of outcomes and complications in 404 stress incontinent women. *International Urogynecology Journal and Pelvic Floor Dysfunction* **Suppl 2**, S24–S27.

Miklos, J. R. (2000). Laparoscopic paravaginal repair plus Burch colposuspension: review and descriptive technique. *Journal of Urology* **56**, 64–69.

Mittleman, R. & Marraccini, J. (1983). Pulmonary Teflon granuloma following periurethral Teflon injection for urinary incontinence. *Archives of Pathology and Laboratory Medicine* **107**, 611–612.

Moehrer, B. *et al.* (2004). Laparoscopic colposuspension for urinary incontinence in women (Cochrane review). In: *The Cochrane Library*, issue 3.

Monga, A. K. *et al.* (1995). Periurethral collagen injection for genuine stress incontinence: a 2 year follow-up. *British Journal of Urology* **76**, 156–170.

Morgan, T. O. *et al.* (2000). Pubovaginal sling: 4 year outcome analysis and quality of life assessment. *Journal of Urology* **163**, 1845–1848.

Nager, C. W. *et al.* (1998). Bulking agents for GSI: short term results and complications in a randomized comparison of periurethral and transurethral injections [abstract]. *Neurourology and Urodynamics* **17**, 314–315.

Nguyen, J. K. & Bhatia, N. N. (2001). Risk of recurrent stress incontinence in women undergoing the combined modified Pereyra procedure and transvaginal sacrospinous ligament vault suspension. *Urology* **58**, 947–952.

Nilsson, C. G. *et al.* (2004). Seven-year follow-up of the tension free vaginal tape procedure for treatment of urinary incontinence. *Obstetrics and Gynaecology* **104**, 1259–1262.

Nilsson, C. G. *et al.* (2001). Long-term results of tension free vaginal tape (TVT) for surgical treatment of female stress urinary incontinence. *International Urogynecology Journal and Pelvic Floor Dysfunction* **12** (Suppl. 2), S5–S8.

O'Connell, H. E. *et al.* (1995). Transurethral collagen therapy in women. *Journal of Urology* **154**, 1463–1465.

Ostrzenski, A. (1998). Genuine stress incontinence in women. New laparoscopic paravaginal reconstruction. *Journal of Reproductive Medicine* **43**, 477–482.

Pannek, J. *et al.* (2001). Particle migration after transurethral injection of carbon coated beads for stress urinary incontinence. *Journal of Urology* **166**, 1350–1353.

Paraiso M. F. R. *et al.* (2004). Laparoscopic Burch colposuspension versus tension-free vaginal tape: a randomised trial. *Obstetrics and Gynecology* **104**, 1249–1258.

Paraiso, M. F. R. *et al.* (1999). Laparoscopic surgery for genuine stress incontinence. *International Urogynecology Journal and Pelvic Floor Dysfunction* **10**, 237–247.

Pelosi II, M. A. *et al.* (2002). The YAMA uropatch sling for treatment of female urinary incontinence: a pilot study. *Journal of Laparoendoscopic and Advanced Surgical Techniques A* **12**, 27–33.

Pereyra, A. J. (1959). A simplified surgical procedure for the correction of stress incontinence in women. *Western Journal of Surgery, Obstetrics and Gynecology* **7**, 223–226.

Persson, J. & Wølner-Hanssen, P. (2000). Laparoscopic Burch Colposuspension for Stress Urinary Incontinence: A Randomized Comparison of One or Two Sutures on Each Side of the Urethra. *Obstetrics & Gynecology* **95**, 151–155.

Petros, P. E. & Ulmsten, U. (1995). Intravaginal slingplasty. An ambulatory surgical procedure for treatment of female urinary stress incontinence. *Scandinavian Journal of Urology, and Nephrology* **29**, 75–82.

Petros, P. E. & Ulmsten, U. (1990). An integral theory of female urinary incontinence. *Acta Obstetricia et Gynecologica Scandinavia* **69** (Suppl. 153), 7–31.

Pickard, R. *et al.* (2004). Periurethral injection therapy for urinary incontinence in women (Cochrane Review). In: *The Cochrane Library*, issue 3.

Quadri, G., Magatti, F., Belloni, C., Barisani, D., Natale, N. (1999). Marshall-Marchetti-Krantz urethropexy and Burch colposuspension for stress urinary incontinence in women with low pressure and hypermobility of the urethra: early results of a prospective randomised clinical trial. *American Journal of Obstetrics and Gynecology* **181**, 12–18.

Radley, S. C. *et al.* (2001). Transurethral implantation of Macroplastique for the treatment of female stress urinary incontinence secondary to urethral sphincter deficiency. *European Urology* **39**, 383–389.

Raldin, C. R. *et al.* (2002a). Tension-free vaginal tape: outcomes among women with primary versus recurrent stress urinary incontinence. *Obstetrics and Gynecology* **100**, 893–897.

Raldin, C. R. *et al.* (2002b). Release of Tension-Free Vaginal Tape for the treatment of refractory postoperative voiding dysfunction. *Obstetrics and Gynecology* **100**, 898–902.

Raz, S. (1981). Modified bladder neck suspension for female stress incontinence. *Urology* **17**, 82–84.

Rechberger, T. *et al.* (2003). A randomised comparison between monofilament and multifilament tapes for stress incontinence surgery. *International Urogynecology Journal and Pelvic Floor Dysfunction* **14**, 432–436.

Rezapour, M. & Ulmsten, U. (2001a). Tension Free Vaginal Tape in women with mixed urinary incontinence. A long term follow-up. *International Urogynecology Journal and Pelvic Floor Dysfunction* **12** (Suppl. 2), S15–S18.

Rezapour M. & Ulmsten U. (2001b). Tension Free Vaginal Tape in women with recurrent stress urinary incontinence. A long term follow-up. *International Urogynecology Journal and Pelvic Floor Dysfunction*, **12** (Suppl. 2), S9–S11.

Richter, H. E. *et al.* (2001). Effects of pubovaginal sling procedure on patients with urethral hypermobility and intrinsic sphincteric deficiency: would they do it again? *American Journal of Obstetrics and Gynecology* **184**, 14–19.

Rothwell, P. (2005). Subgroup analysis in randomised controlled trials: importance, indications, and interpretation. *Lancet* **365**, 176–186.

Saidi, M. H. *et al.* (1998). Extraperitoneal laparoscopic colposuspension: short-term cure rate, complications, and duration of hospital stay in comparison with Burch colposuspension. *Obstetrics and Gynaecology* **92**, 619–621.

Santarosa, R. P. *et al.* (1994). Periurethral injection of autologous fat for the treatment of sphincteric incontinence. *Journal of Urology* **151**, 607–611.

Scotti, R. J. *et al.* (1998). Paravaginal repair of vaginal wall defects by fixation to the ischial periosteum and obturator membrane. *American Journal of Obstetrics and Gynecology* **179**, 1436–1445.

Segal, J. L. *et al.* (2004). Prevalence of persistent and de novo overactive bladder symptoms after the tension-free vaginal tape. *Obstetrics and Gynecology* **104**, 1263–1269.

Sheriff, M. K. M. *et al.* (1997). Endoscopic correction of intractable stress incontinence with silicone micro-implants. *European Urology* **32**, 284–288.

Shull, B. L. & Baden, W. F. (1989). A six years experience with paravaginal defects repair for stress urinary incontinence. *American Journal of Obstetrics and Gynecology* **160**, 1432–1439.

Smith, D. N. *et al.* (1997). Collagen injection therapy for female intrinsic sphincter deficiency. *Journal of Urology* **157**, 1275–1278.

Stamey, T. A. (1973). Endoscopic suspension of vesical neck for urinary incontinence. *Surgery, Gynecology and Obstetrics* **136**, 547–548.

Stothers, L. *et al.* (1998). Complications of periurethral collagen injection for stress urinary incontinence. *Journal of Urology* **159**, 806–807.

Su, T. H. *et al.* (1998). Periurethral fat injection in the treatment of recurrent genuine stress incontinence. *Journal of Urology* **159**, 411–414.

Su, T. H. *et al.* (1997). Prospective comparison of traditional colposuspensions in the treatment of genuine stress incontinence. *Acta Obstetricia et Gynecologica Scandinavica* **6**, 576–582.

Summitt, R. L. *et al.* (2000). Randomised comparison of laparoscopic and transabdominal Burch urethropexy for the treatment of genuine stress incontinence. *Obstetrics and Gynecology* **95** (4 Suppl. 1): S2.

Swami S. *et al.* (1997). Collagen for female genuine stress incontinence after a minimum 2 year follow-up. *Journal of Urology* **80**, 757–761.

Tamanini, J. T. N. *et al.* (2003). Macroplastique implantation system for the treatment of female stress urinary incontinence. *Journal of Urology* **169**, 2229–2233.

Tamussino, K. *et al.* (2001a). The Austrian tension-free vaginal tape registry. *International Urogynecology Journal and Pelvic Floor Dysfunction* 12 (Suppl. 2), S28–S29.

Tamussino, K. *et al.* (2001b). Tension-free vaginal tape operation: results of the Austrian registry. *Obstetrics and Gynaecology* **98**, 732–736.

Tamussino, K. F. *et al.* (1999). Five years results after anti-incontinence operations. *American Journal of Obstetrics and Gynecology* **181**, 1347–1352.

Tayrac, R. *et al.* (2002). Comparison of anterior colporrhaphy versus Bologna procedure in women with genuine stress incontinence. *International Urogynecology Journal and Pelvic Floor Dysfunction* **13**, 36–39.

Takahashi, S. *et al.* (2002). Complications of Stamey needle suspension for female stress urinary incontinence. *Urology International* **68**, 148–151.

Takar, R. *et al.* (2002). Secondary colposuspension: results of a prospective study from a tertiary referral centre. *British Journal of Obstetrics and Gynecology* **109**, 115–120.

Tebyani, N. *et al.* (2000). Percutaneous needle bladder neck suspension for the treatment of stress urinary incontinence in women: long-term results. *Journal of Urology* **163**, 1510–1512.

Trokman, B. A. *et al.* (1995). Surgical treatment of intrinsic urethral dysfunction: injectables (fat). *Urologic Clinics of North America* **22**, 655–671.

Tsivian, A. *et al.* (2004). Tape related complications of the tension-free vaginal tape procedure. *Journal of Urology* **171**, 762–764.

Tsivian, A. *et al.* (2003). Bone-anchor 4-corner cystourethropexy: long term results. *Journal of Urology* **169**, 2244–2245.

Ulmsten, U. *et al.* (1999). A three year follow-up of TVT for surgical treatment of female stress incontinence. *British Journal of Obstetrics and Gynecology* **106**, 345–350.

Usman, F. & Henalla, S. (1998). A single macroplastique injection as primary treatment for stress incontinence in women. *Journal of Obstetrics and Gynecology* **18**, 56–60.

Ustun, Y. *et al.* (2003). Tension free vaginal tape compared with laparoscopic Burch urethropexy. *Journal of the American Association of Gynecologic Laparoscopist* **10**, 386–389.

Valpas, A. *et al.* (2004). Tension-free vaginal tape and laparoscopic mesh colposuspension for stress urinary incontinence. *Obstetrics and Gynecology* **104**, 42–49.

Valpas, A. *et al.* (2003). Tension-free vaginal tape and laparoscopic mesh colposuspension in the treatment of stress urinary incontinence: immediate outcome and complications. A randomised clinical trial. *Acta Obstetricia and Gynecologica Scandinavica* **82**, 665–671.

Vancaille, T. G. & Schussler, W. (1991). Laparoscopic bladder neck suspension. *Journal of Laparoendoscopic Surgery* **1**, 169–173.

Vierek, V. *et al.* (2004). Introital ultrasound of the lower genital tract before and after colposuspension: a 4 year objective follow up. *Ultrasound Obstetrics and Gynecology* **23**, 277–283.

Vierhout, M. E. (2001). Severe haemorrhage complicating tension free vaginal tape (TVT): a case report. *International Urogynecology Journal and Pelvic Floor Dysfunction* **12**, 139–140.

Walsh, I. K. *et al.* (2002). Cadaveric fascia lata pubovaginal sling: early results on safety, efficacy and patient satisfaction. *British Journal of Urology* **90**, 415–419.

Wang, K. H. *et al.* (2003). Comparison of tension-free vaginal tapping versus modified Burch colposuspension on urethral obstruction: a randomised controlled trial. *Neurourology and Urodynamics* **22**, 185–190.

Wang, K. H. *et al.* (2002). Voiding dysfunction following TVT procedure. *International Urogynecology Journal and Pelvic Floor Dysfunction* **13**, 353–358.

Ward, K & Hilton, P. (2002). Prospective multicentre randomised trial of tension free vaginal tape and colposuspension as primary treatment for stress incontinence. *British Medical Journal* **325**, 67–73.

Ward, K & Hilton, P. (2004). A prospective multi-centre randomised trial of tension-free vaginal tape and colposuspension for primary urodynamic stress incontinence: two-year follow-up. *American Journal of Obstetrics and Gynecology* **190**, 324–331.

Wennberg, A. L. *et al.* (2003). Stamey's abdomino-vaginal needle colposuspension for the correction of female genuine stress urinary incontinence. Long-term results. *Scandinavian Journal of Urology and Nephrology* **37**, 419–423.

White, C. (1909). Cystocoele. *Journal of the American Medical Association* **21**, 1707–1710.

Winters, J. C. *et al.* (1995). Periurethral injection of collagen in the treatment of intrinsic sphincteric deficiency in the female patient. *Urologic Clinics of North America* **148**, 1797–1800.

Wright, E. J. *et al.* (1998). Pubovaginal sling using cadaveric allograft fascia for the treatment of intrinsic sphincter deficiency. *Journal of Urology* **160**, 759–762.

Zaragoza, M. R. *et al.* (1996). Expanded indications for pubovaginal sling: treatment of Type 2 or 3 stress incontinence. *Journal of Urology* **156**, 1620–1622.

Zilberg, A. W. & Farrell, S. A. (2001). External iliac artery laceration during tension-free vaginal tape procedure. *International Urogynecology Journal and Pelvic Floor Dysfunction* **12**, 141–143.

Zullo, F. *et al.* (2001). Laparoscopic Burch colposuspension: a randomized controlled trial comparing two transperitoneal surgical techniques. *Obstetrics and Gynecology* **98**, 783–789.

PART 4

Service development and evaluation

Chapter 12

What is effective in the development and management of integrated continence services?

Judith Wardle

Background

The concept of integrated continence services was first expounded in detail in the Department of Health guidance document *Good Practice in Continence Services* (March 2000), although there are earlier references to the concept of comprehensive services, for instance in *Commissioning Comprehensive Continence Services* by Christine Norton (Norton 1995). Unfortunately, the Department's document had no regulatory force, much to the disappointment of the Working Party chaired by Professor Paul Abrams. Also, despite its title, it contained no examples of individual good practice in the field, which could have provided models for the development of services around the country. (Such examples could have been provided, but the Department chose to produce a document stronger on theory than practical information.)

As one way of redressing the absence of information that could be used to plan improved services, the Continence Foundation, with input from the other continence charities, published *Making the Case for Investment in an Integrated Continence Service* (Pollock 2000). This document contains prevalence information and advice on how to calculate the number of people affected in a given area, taking account of such factors as the number of nursing homes and the presence of ethnic minorities. It gives brief advice on the impact on quality of life with references to documents that set out evidence for practices that are clinically effective. Possibly the most significant section for influencing the development of services was that entitled 'The cost of incontinence in the NHS.' Surprisingly, the Department had never worked out what incontinence was costing the NHS. In an effort to provide a preliminary estimate of these costs, David Pollock, then Director of the Continence Foundation, reviewed an extensive number of articles and documents relating to the costs of drugs, appliances, containment products, staff costs and surgery in the hope that such data would provide continence services with the necessary arguments to try to persuade their local Primary Care Groups (as they were then termed) that developing a more integrated service was not only in the interests of staff and patients, but might also be cost-effective.

The Foundation additionally set out to ensure that the innovative ideas on integrated services that had been advanced were actively considered by the Department. Indeed, when a Parliamentary Question placed in June 2000 asking whether the Department of Health intended to monitor the implementation of the Guidance was answered in the negative, the Foundation and The Royal College of Nursing's Continence Care Forum set about designing their own two-year research project to find out whether there had been 'significant change in continence services provision' following publication of the Guidance. Funding was obtained from the PPP Foundation and Sue Thomas, policy and practice adviser at The Royal College of Nursing, led the research programme assisted by continence advisers and a statistician. The Continence Foundation provided a Steering Group to contribute to the design of questionnaires and to the organisation of local events to run in parallel with the research. In addition, the Foundation also organised two national conferences to publicise examples of good practice identified during the research or identified as a result of other enquiries. The main research took place over two years so that the pace of change could be monitored. It covered all primary care organisations in five of the then eight Health Authorities of England and was conducted via two questionnaires addressed to continence advisors and the lead person within the Trust, with a follow-up telephone call to ensure that all aspects of the questionnaires were understood. Response rate in the first year was 75% and in the second year was 68%. The following first and second year reports on the research are available from the Continence Foundation: *Good, Better, Best Practice* and *Is Policy Translated into Action?* (Thomas 2002, 2003). To bring the data generated by this research up to date, a brief follow-up questionnaire was sent out by the author of this chapter in November 2004 by e-mail to leads of continence services and distributed to attendees at a conference of the RCN Continence Care Forum – it is recognised that the method of administering this questionnaire would give a bias towards the most committed services.

The Department of Health eventually redressed its initial failure to set a target date for the creation of integrated services: this appeared in the National Service Framework for Older People (DoH 2001b): milestones attached to Standard 2, Person-centred care, required plans for such a service to be detailed by primary care organisations by April 2003 and to be implemented by April 2004.

What constitutes an Integrated Continence Service?

There are two ways of describing an integrated continence service:

1. By setting out the activities performed in relation to the relevant population that together add up to a continuum of care;
2. By listing the professionals, departments and Authorities that need to relate easily with each other to the same end.

Thanks to our supporters,
Cancer Research UK is able
to fund more research into
the causes and treatments
of children's cancers than
any other UK organisation.
This work is saving
children's lives.

- In the 1960s, only
  one in four children
  survived cancer.

- Now, the number of
  children surviving cancer
  is three out of four.

To learn more about
the work of
Cancer Research UK
please visit
www.cancerresearchuk.org

**It's a sign of hope for
children with cancer.**

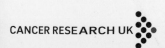

CANCER RESEARCH UK

A
thank you
at
Christmas

Your support has
given children and their
families the gift of hope
this Christmas.

Such generosity
means that more
children will be able
to survive cancer, and
enjoy the magic of
the festive season.

Thank you.

Keeping the two aspects separate helps to make it clear that the first of these can be defined on a national basis (and perhaps international): this is the pathway of care needed to meet clinical and social standards. The second is more subject to variation according to what degrees of skill and what specialities are available at a local level and how services are configured within a region.

Extrapolating from the Guidance, the elements of service need to cover:

- raising awareness among the public and health professionals
- identification of incontinent individuals and those at risk
- initial assessment of individuals
- a management or treatment plan (including a timetable for review) agreed with the individual and/or carer
- referral, if appropriate, to more specialist services, which will perform more detailed assessment and carry out treatment.

The next step in the process is not mentioned in the Guidance: referral back to less specialist services for ongoing management or treatment. For the most part, this step does take place, but I mention it because we hear of people who fail to receive the necessary follow-up. The Guidance also omits to mention discharge from the service for people who have been successfully treated.

The providers of continence services are, self-evidently, based in primary, secondary and tertiary tiers of the health service. This suggests the triangular representation of the service which has been so much used recently in Departmental documents as an image of the needs of people with long-term conditions and provision for their needs. However, the hierarchical implication of that image cannot be allowed to work against the new flexibility of roles which is occurring within the nursing and caring professions. Moreover, we also need an image to take account of the input needed from authorities other than health. Health Trusts (primary and acute) need to work with social services, both in the community and in care homes, and with education authorities – the Guidance picks up on both of these; and for some, there will be a need for liaison with providers of housing or transport – such factors are emphasized by anyone with an interest in long-term conditions. It is also important not to ignore the role of the independent sector, most obviously providers of care homes and support services, but also pharmacists whose role is increasing under their new contract and the manufacturers of medicines, containment products and diagnostic devices.

It is important that there is a breadth of service provision as well as all levels of speciality. Client groups who might miss getting an equitable service include people with learning disabilities, mental health problems, physical disabilities or neurological problems. The service must encompass all age groups: organisation of services for children or older people might be partly separate but must be equitable and there must be smooth transitions with adult services. The Guidance also refers to other people who might be disadvantaged: ethnic minorities, travellers, asylum seekers and refugees, prisoners and those suffering socio-economic disadvantage. It is axiomatic that there should be the same quality of service for men and women and for both urinary and faecal problems.

For an integrated service to be developed and to function, there also need to be organisational elements. The Guidance specified a 'Director' of continence services for groups of primary care organisations. The fact that the title has met with resistance does not alter the need to have a person or persons with this strategic role. The description in the Guidance of the role of a director is a good summary of the strategic elements that must be in place. Thus, someone needs to be responsible for:

- overseeing and co-ordinating the development and implementation of common policies, procedures and protocols
- developing and maintaining care pathways to and from primary care and specialist services
- ensuring users and carers are involved in all aspects of the service
- working closely with other services such as social services, education services and psychological services
- ensuring services are made available to all patients in hospital who require them
- co-ordinating educational activities for continence specialists, primary health care teams and others involved in the delivery of health and social care
- organising service-wide review, audit and research activities particularly to ensure national targets are met
- promoting awareness of continence (Guidance, p. 14).

What progress had been made?

In 2002, 56% of respondents had plans to develop an integrated service; by 2003 this had increased to 91% (Thomas 2003). However, a survey by the Director of the Continence Foundation (this author) in November 2004 found only three areas claiming to have achieved an integrated service, six more were expecting to complete by April 2005 or soon after and a further five within the year – note that because integrated services will be created by groups of PCTs (and some Acute Trusts) it is only possible to approximate what the total number might be. However, based on four Trusts per integrated service, this would constitute about a fifth of the services in England (some services in Wales and Scotland are working to a similar model, even though they are not subject to the Guidance.)

A principal concern remains the lack of support for the strategic work required. The title of 'Director' is not necessary to achieve leadership: about half of services have an individual who has adopted a leadership role. However, some colleagues recognise that responsibilies have fallen to them by default rather than intention and they may therefore not feel confident in their role. Most valuable characteristics in a service that is moving rapidly towards integration are drive and assertiveness, but such personalities need time to develop. To be effective, the colleague who has adopted a leadership role needs to be supported in that role: only three such individuals had been appointed at the time of writing specifically to create integration; few colleagues have protected time (an example that may be cited is the continence team in Gloucestershire, which happens to be based in an Acute Trust, and which has been able to make the decision to redesign operational roles to free up some time for one person to engage in strategic work); and few have a specific budget for the work – clearly impracticable. Not enough strategic planning is therefore taking place: the Leeds service had the excellent idea, for example, of creating both a strategy and an operations group, so that these two aspects did not become confused in the same meeting.

Support also needs to come from Board level. While half have managed to get discussions at PCT Board level (up from a third in 2003), only a third of Local Development Plans mention integrated continence services (no change from the previous year). Moreover, a search of the internet found only two Strategic Health Authority reports that mention the subject – West Midlands and Dorset & Somerset.

What factors do services that are close to integration have in common?

As has been emphasized, PCTs need to work together in groups: one PCT will take the lead and have a Service Level Agreement with the others, thus creating sufficient population and budget to provide for specialisms: one PCT could not have the resources to provide continence advisors with special knowledge of, for instance, children, men, mental health, or ethnic minorities. The most innovative services encompass four to six Trusts, mainly PCTs, but some have included Acute Trusts or Trusts for mental health or learning disability. Logic suggests that including secondary level personnel should dispel tensions that might arise between them and staff from primary care, but as yet there is no research information available to support such an assertion. Another very new development that may be advantageous is the closer collaboration of health and social services in a few areas into a partnership body, for example, South Essex. The population range is from 400,000 to one Million; clearly, geography is a factor in the decision on how large the group can be.

All relevant nurse or physiotherapy specialists and consultants in secondary care need to have some involvement in the planning of the service. These should include urodynamics services, nurses on acute wards, a urologist, a gynaecologist, a geriatrician, a gastroenterologist, a dietician and a paediatrician. Where tertiary specialisms such as urogynaecology, coloproctology or neurology are in the same hospital as the secondary services, it would be advantageous to seek their input. One service (South Essex) is also known to be planning to include palliative care services in their arrangements.

Possible barriers to the achievement of integrated continence services

It is difficult to persuade PCT Boards to take an interest in continence among so many competing priorities. It has always been difficult to stimulate interest in the condition in more than a small number of general practitioners and this task becomes even more difficult with the advent of the new GP contracts. In some instances, barriers are created by individuals who are concerned about possible loss of their own status within a system which involves a blurring of boundaries between roles and freeing up referral systems. The most difficult organisations to bring within the frame of an integrated service will be the large teaching hospitals, which by definition have relationships with a wide range of other acute and primary trusts and may have less contact with social care.

One element proposed for an integrated service which appears to have created difficulties is the involvement of users and carers in 'the planning, provision and audit of services' (Guidance 3.2). *Essence of Care*, the 2001 document on the principles of benchmarking, separated standards relating to users of continence services into two elements: 'patient to patient support actively promoted' and 'Users are always involved in planning and evaluating services, and their input is acted upon' (Department of Health 2001a). The provision of patient to patient support is available in about a third of services via some form of user group, either set up by the continence advisors or working with the charity, *In*Contact.

Much more difficult is devising ways to involve users at a strategic level. Including a token user on a strategy group is unlikely to ensure that planning meets the needs of the most vulnerable groups. Some services have involved users in specific aspects of service redesign and this appears to be effective: while involving users in audit of products provision will have only a small impact, more innovative ideas include inviting patients to sessions of process mapping, having a patient on an interview panel for new staff, using questionnaires during the planning process to obtain the views of a wider range of users and tapping into local Patient Forums, some of which are gaining expertise in understanding planning issues for a variety of medical conditions. Perhaps the greatest problem is the 'unevenness' of development of integrated continence services across the country. There is no doubt that there will be several excellent services operating, even if there are variations in the model. However, at the other extreme, there are services within one PCT which are operated by a single continence advisor who is too busy with clinical commitments even to think about strategic developments. With a few notable exceptions, the impetus to move towards integration has come from continence advisors who have developed good interpersonal skills as well as having dogged determination. The challenge is to find ways to bring the most isolated services up to the highest standards and to import strategic skills from elsewhere to enable this change to take place.

Examples of elements essential to an integrated service that have been successfully implemented in some areas

Uniform assessment forms and care pathways

Care Pathways that include assessment tools are an essential component of the primary and secondary element of an integrated service. Ideally, these should be available in electronic format so that each person providing identification and assessment of continence problems contributes as much as their knowledge permits, with the result being communicated to a colleague with more specialist knowledge to complete any missing sections. Such systems should also include a 'red flag' system to ensure that anyone with symptoms that require urgent treatment is referred immediately to the appropriate consultant. There is no reason why such care pathways cannot be uniform throughout the country, not just within a particular area.

Care Pathways have long been in operation within the NHS, and possible local variations have been identified by disseminating these tools widely with the Continence Care Forum and then collating suggestions. They cover both urinary and faecal symptoms (Bayliss et al. 2003). Further development might be possible in secondary care: they have been adopted by several hospitals, but there is so far no uniformity about the additional elements.

Making referral systems more logical

Dudley PCT was fortunate to have a GP who demonstrated an interest in incontinence. This colleague may be identified as Dr John Firth who acts as a clinical assistant in uro-gynaecology at the University Hospital Birmingham. In 1994, a multi-disciplinary team consisting of a public health registrar, a continence advisor, a physiotherapist, community nurses, a gynaecologist, a urologist and a GP, published a care pathway to preclude inappropriate gynaecological referrals. For example, patients who did not, as claimed, have stress incontinence, but who did have bladder dysfunction. The consequence of inappropriate referrals was wasted time for both gynaecologist and patient, since the patient would then be referred back to the GP, the physiotherapist or for urodynamics. Also, the skills of continence advisors and physiotherapists were being under-utilized, and gynaecology nurses were keen to learn and conduct urodynamic assessments.

So, Dr Firth, the GP to whom this author refers, generated a care pathway that would also include health visitors (since these workers have the ability to identify symptoms of incontinence in the first place) two nurses working in the hospital, and a midwife with skills in audit. Where patients did present first to him, he would take a history and carry out a physical examination and urinalysis to rule out conditions that did require urgent referral to a consultant, but otherwise the patient's next referral was to a continence adviser. Other people might self-refer to the continence adviser, be referred from the community or by hospital staff. The continence advisers were using the same criteria for urgent referral to a consultant, and importantly the same paperwork so that investigations were not repeated. Continence advisers ensured that lifestyle modification and conservative treatments were considered, involving physiotherapists or occupational therapists as required, advising the GP where treatment was successful or referring the patient to the GP for further investigation. As Dr Firth stated when making a presentation at the Continence Foundation's conference in October 2002, 'the theory is fine, but it is difficult to actually make it work ... it tends to be letters that do the rounds rather than the patient' (Firth 2002).

Tracking the patient journey/process mapping

More detailed analysis of the consequences of local referral practices has been conducted to study service deficiencies and identify opportunities for quality improvements. A project was designed by the Integrated Continence Forum of the service which is now based in East Elmbridge & Mid Surrey PCT (formerly part of an acute/community Trust) to analyse the patient journey for females with urinary incontinence. Rowena Lavender, who was the senior continence advisor, reported that the initial process involved 'brown paper, post-it notes, honesty and humour'. (Recently, software has been developed for 'process mapping' which not only enables the detailing of what actions need to come in what order, but also who is responsible for each stage and this methodology may well initiate change.) Out of the analysis came a diagram of how complex the client journey might be (Figure 12.1).

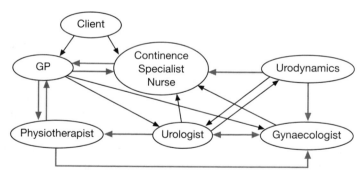

Figure 12.1 The appointment system

Some patients who could have benefited from conservative treatment were identified as having been referred immediately for surgery and it seemed clear that they were receiving inadequate information with which to make decisions, having implications not only for the patient but also the NHS.

Important to the success of the project was the setting of clear aims and outcome measures. The work also enhanced the function of the Integrated Continence Forum, especially once a consultant with an interest in female urology had been appointed and charitable funds were found for additional physiotherapy training. The improvement in the efficiency of the pathway is illustrated in Figure 12.2.

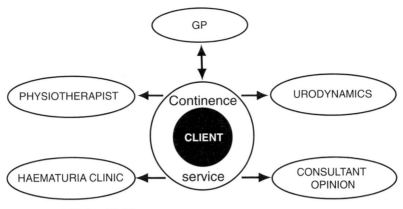

Source: Lavender & Walker (2003).

Figure 12.2 Modification of the patient referral system following implementation of quality improvements

Providing training to non-specialists to facilitate identification of continence problems

There are several examples of work that takes account of the aspiration of non-specialists to develop their skills while increasing the pool of people able to contribute to continence services.

In the Ribble Valley, it was recognised that District or Practice Nurses were often the 'gateway' into continence services and that they might already have a relationship with potential patients via screening programmes or via initial contracts for other medical problems. Therefore, it was logical to seek to develop their skills so that they could recognise continence problems and initiate treatment. These colleagues were also encouraged to provide patient education on the subject. Training given in pelvic floor examination, use of a bladder scanner and knowledge of secondary care procedures, meant that they could initiate basic treatment, advise GPs and refer appropriately to consultants, this last function requiring changes in policy and practice with improvements being documented in the efficiency of clinical services (Hill 2002).

Employing essentially similar principles, colleagues operating the continence service in Nottingham City decided that they needed to work more closely with social services and to develop the skills of staff in nursing homes: the project started was initiated due to serious concerns about continence assessment and management within a particular nursing home. Better trained nurses within this and other homes have been able to institute continence management programmes as well as to make appropriate decisions about containment products. Further development of this training programme was aided by the shift in responsibility for all care homes to the NHS, since 'funded' nursing care brought additional cost pressures. This particular service was able to obtain an F grade nurse to support this work.

Moving assessment further into the community, the Nottingham continence service developed clinics in day centres. The change in attitudes created by having a clinic in a day centre for older people with mental health problems persuaded Social Services initially to fund two grade G nursing posts, and these posts were eventually funded by joint health and social care monies. It was recognised that a continence service in day centres could maintain people in their own homes for longer periods. As the service evolved across the area to include people with learning and physical disabilities, it became apparent that nurses working in outreach clinics required a portable bladder scanner. Important to the success of the project was the recognition of the need to include secretarial support in the bid for funding since it is axiomatic that it is a poor use of resources for grade G nurses to be occupied with administration. Also important was the inclusion of outcome measures in all bids for funding so that evidence of value for money would become available.

Nottingham is one of the areas in the UK which hopes to have a fully integrated continence service before many others. The final design will include several joint clinics between continence advisors and consultants, liaison with mental health and learning disability services as well as work with social services and a clinic in a multiple sclerosis centre. Final improvements to the service will relate to faecal incontinence (Brown 2003).

Most services which are moving towards integration now offer training to district and practice nurses, health visitors and staff in care homes and a few also offer training to midwives.

Materials available to assist with creating integrated services

As part of its commitment to disseminate information about examples of good practice in various aspects of an integrated service, the Continence Foundation has made available CDs of the presentations and workshops at its two national conferences 'Integrated Continence Services: Good Better Best Practice' (2002) and 'Integrated Continence Services: Making it Happen!' (2003). The Children's Continence Action Group worked together to produce indicators and examples of best practice regarding a paediatric service for the eleven factors for benchmarking of continence services in Chapter 7 of the *Essence of Care*. The Association for Continence Advice has produced a folder, *Steps 2 Success: the Toolkit for Multi-Professional Continence Care* (ACA 2004). This contains a variety of advice and templates for developing the various skills required in primary care. The only material available that comprehensively examines the concept of an integrated service and focuses on the strategic level is a folder of documents and a CD produced in 2003 by the Continence Foundation. This has the same title as the Foundation's 2002 conference, *Integrated Continence Services: Good, Better, and Best Practice*. It was formulated by Thomas and Wardle (Thomas & Wardle 2003). Of particular significance is the document available on the CD, so that users can enter details of their local service. Its title is 'A strategic framework for implementing Good Practice in Continence Services.' There are at the time of writing no published articles which comprehensively address the design of integrated continence services other than brief communications.

What still needs to be done

The few services that have already achieved an integrated service or are well on the way to achievement have yet to provide the outcome data that is needed to convince other PCTs and Strategic Health Authorities that such a service is both economically viable and in the interests of all patients. Of course, to progress to that point, they will have convinced their local commissioners of the need for integration. What is now needed are data from a systematic audit which demonstrate clear improvements and associated cost benefits.

One area which will certainly be producing outcome data is Gwent. This service, in Wales UK, is operated by a Nurse Consultant in Continence and has been at the forefront of the development of integrated continence services (Logan & Proctor 2003). Services in England will be auditing themselves as part of The Royal College of Physicians project led by Dr Adrian Wagg. Services at the forefront of developing integration need to be encouraged to extend their auditing to the entire service and to publish the results so that these can be used as evidence for developments elsewhere. Otherwise, the 'postcode lottery' for people in need of continence services, which was identified by the Guidance as existing in 2000, may extend into all aspects of continence provision.

References

Bayliss, V. *et al.* (2003). Pathways for continence care: an audit to assess how they are used. *British Journal of Nursing* **12**(14) 857–863.

Brown, S. (2003). *Building an Integrated Continence Service.* Aylesbury: Diagnostic Ultrasound.

Continence Foundation (2002). *Integrated Continence Services: Good, Better and Best Practice.*

Continence Foundation (2003). *Integrated Continence Services: Making it Happen!*

Department of Health (2000). *Good Practice in Continence Services.* London.

Department of Health (2001a). *Essence of Care: Patient-focused Benchmarking for Health Care Practitioners.* London.

Department of Health (2001b). *National Service Framework for Older People.* London.

Firth, J. (2002). *A Care Pathway from Primary Care.* Presentation on Continence Foundation CD.

Hill, S. (2002). *Developing the role of District Nurses in continence management: Breaking down barriers.* Presentation on Continence Foundation CD.

Lavender, R. & Walker, R. (2003). Simplifying the client journey for females with urinary incontinence. *Clinical Governance Bulletin* **4**, 6–8.

Logan, K. & Proctor, S. (2003). Developing an interdisciplinary integrated continence service. *Nursing Times, 27* May – 2 Jun; **99** (21), 34–37.

Norton, C. (1995). *Commissioning Comprehensive Continence Services*, London: Continence Foundation.

Pollock, D. (2000). *Making the Case for Integrated Continence Services: A Source Book for Continence Services*. London: Continence Foundation.

Thomas, S. (2002). *Good, Better, Best Practice*. London: Continence Foundation.

Thomas, S (2003). *Is Policy Translated into Action?* London: Continence Foundation and The Royal College of Nursing.

Thomas, S. & Wardle, J. (2003). *Integrated Continence Services: Good, Better and Best Practice*. London: Continence Foundation.

Chapter 13

Government targets, audit data and outcome indicators in the measurement of clinical performance

Adrian Wagg

Introduction

In 1999, the UK Government published *A First Class Service: Quality in the New NHS* (Department of Health 1998a) that set out a framework for quality improvement and fair access to services within the NHS. There had been a series of 'scandals' within the organisation and a realisation that the public were more questioning of professionals and services than had previously been the case. This document proposed three elements to ensure high-quality care: clear national standards for services and treatments, through National Service Frameworks and the National Institute for Clinical Excellence (NICE), local delivery of high-quality health care through clinical governance and effective monitoring of progress via the Commission for Health Improvement. Essentially, these basic tenets still exist although there has been organisational change in the intervening years and the monitoring of the implementation of clinical guidelines and audit has been taken on by the Healthcare Commission and NICE. In reality, clinical guidelines and clinical, or medical, audit and production of guidelines predated what is now known as clinical governance. The processes to improve the quality of health care services provision have been in place for many years. Although the terms and language used to describe these processes have, over time, changed, the task remains the same. Clinical governance is the latest in a long list of such changes. This article deals with quality indicators, their use in the field of urinary incontinence and mechanisms by which change might be achieved.

Quality indicators and guidelines: measurement

Clinical indicators and audit tools derived from evidence-based guidelines have been developed for urinary incontinence (Working Group on Outcome Indicators for Urinary Incontinence 1997; Button *et al.* 1998; Cheater *et al.* 1998). Clinical or outcome indicators are aggregated statistical measures that describe either a group of patients or a population and provide pointers to the quality of care without necessarily being directly related to quality. Outcome indicators have, therefore, been refined over the years to be more directly related to outcomes and to describe the underlying quality of care, either good or deficient, to allow judgements to be made from the results of data collection. Indicators cover the organisation of care, (structure), the clinical process of care and the outcomes from that care. In addition, indicators have been developed that cover case finding and aspects of preventative measures against the development of incontinence.

The National Centre for Health Outcomes Development (NCHOD) used a specialist panel of experts to define 18 clinical indicators to measure the quality of care with regard to urinary incontinence which covered all areas of care, including avoiding the risk of incontinence, the reduction of delays in assessment, for treatment of the underlying diagnoses and associated quality of life measures (Brocklehurst *et al.* 1999). This detailed report set out the population of patients for which the guidelines were relevant, the data sources to enable collection of the data and recommended how regularly the items might be collected to be clinically useful. In 1998, The Royal College of Physicians Research Unit completed a pilot assessment of three of the NCHOD indicators that were relevant to older people in long-term care settings. The results demonstrated that the clinical indicators (such as the number of individuals with indwelling catheters, or prevalence of incontinence) were of benefit to individual units, but required further refinement before being adopted for comparisons between units (Georgiou *et al.* 2001). The Royal College of Physicians also developed the Continuous Assessment Review and Evaluation scheme, a clinical audit package for long-term care for older people which included a continence module and a separate continence audit tool (Research Unit, Royal College of Physicians of London 1998; Royal College of Physicians of London 1998). The Department of Health publication *Good Practice in Continence Services* (Department of Health 2000) identified great variance in the quality of and access to continence services and acknowledged that although many incontinent individuals were likely to be in contact with either their health or social services, these services were unlikely to be aware of their problem. The aim of this review was to ensure the nationwide availability of high-quality services for people with incontinence and to set clear and achievable targets for service. The document covered all areas of care, setting targets for primary, secondary and continuing care (Figure 13.1). The guidance also included recommendations for the conduct of clinical audit and set standards to which management might be compared. Unfortunately, the content of this document, which was originally intended to mandate action on the part of the health service, was downgraded to the level of 'voluntary recommendation' due to 'target overload ' from the Department of Health at the time of publication and thus progress for continence services has been slow.

There is evidence from other conditions demonstrating that clinical indicators can be used to measure the quality of care and to influence the assessment and management of conditions, leading to an improvement in the care delivered to patients. The National Sentinel Audit of Stroke has been successful in demonstrating the variation in standards of care in hospitals around the country and the improvement

NHS Trusts should ensure that:

- Effective surgical procedures for incontinence are undertaken and that they are carried out by surgeons who do an adequate volume to maintain their expertise and achieve good outcomes for their patients.

- Patients, newly presenting in hospital with incontinence, are identified, properly assessed and managed.

- Patients in NHS continuing care facilities with incontinence are identified, assessed and appropriately managed and treated.

- Proactive steps are taken to identify patients with incontinence problems that might arise after treatment.

Figure 13.1 Targets for NHS Trusts. From Good Practice in Continence Services (Department of Health 2000)

that can be achieved with feedback to individual sites (Irwin *et al.* 2005). Within primary care, measurement of key clinical indicators has demonstrated improvements in management of hypertension, diabetes and asthma in association with the application of guidelines (Feder *et al.* 1995; Cranney *et al.* 1999). Building on its previous work, the Clinical Effectiveness and Evaluation Unit of the Royal College of Physicians has completed a two-year programme that aimed to develop and refine quality indicators for urinary and faecal incontinence in older people, although many of these are not age specific. The experience gained from piloting the NCHOD indicators was used to refine the then available indicators from all of the available sources in 2001. Where there were no indicators in a defined area, standard methods (consensus workshops/Delphi panels) were used to identify additional clinical indicators that might be used and that might be directly related to patient care. It was intended that the indicators developed would be piloted to establish their use on a national basis in order to measure the quality of care with regard to incontinence, to demonstrate the degree of variability in the quality of care and to be used as a basis for improving the quality of care. The indicators were primarily aimed at the care received by older people (> 65 years) in order to meet the needs of the National Service Framework for Older People (2001). In addition *The New NHS: Modern and Dependable* (Department of Health 1998b) sought to reduce variation in the standards of care around the country and to drive up the standards of care. The development of the National Service Framework for Older People (2001) included task groups considering the dignity of patients, carer strain and transitions of care, all issues that are particularly relevant to urinary and faecal incontinence. However, the only action mandated by this document was the establishment of integrated continence services for older people by April 2004, a target that has been almost universally missed

(Thomas 2003). The importance of incontinence as a functional diagnosis in long-term care settings was highlighted by The Royal College of Physicians joint report on the health and care of older people in care homes (Royal College of Physicians of London 2000). There is also a pressing economic need to pay attention to this costly area of care.

The publication of *Essence of Care* by The Royal College of Nursing included continence as a key area of its work and emphasised the need for privacy and dignity in providing care to patients with a potentially embarrassing problem. The document set out standards for what is termed benchmarking (essentially a comparative clinical audit) in continence care (Royal College of Nursing 2000).

The output of the Cochrane collaboration may also be used as a source of evidence-based guidelines in areas of continence care. Thus far, amongst other areas, the collaboration has considered bladder retraining (Wallace *et al.* 2005), behavioural therapies (Hay-Smith 2003) and prompted voiding (Eustice *et al.* 2005), in addition to a variety of surgical procedures for stress urinary incontinence (http://www.updatesoftware.com/search/search.asp?zoom_query=incontinence&zoom_page=3&zoom_per_page=10&zoom_cat=-1&zoom_and=0: accessed 8 August 2005). The deliberation of the committees of the International Consultation on Incontinence may also be used as a source of expert consensus from which to draw indicators of the quality of care for people with urinary incontinence (Abrams *et al.* 2005). Guidelines from the European Association of Urology essentially follow the same lines and are produced as flow diagrams (Hampel *et al.* 1999). The American Agency for Health Care Policy and Research (AHCPR) released its first guideline on urinary incontinence in 1992. This guideline is now obsolete and has not been reissued but is still a valuable guideline for the generation of quality standards (AHCPR 1996).

In addition to the existing guidelines, the Scottish Intercollegiate Guidelines Network have published guidelines for the management of urinary incontinence in primary care, and, for England, Wales and Northern Ireland, NICE have embarked upon the production of clinical guidelines for the treatment of urinary incontinence and prolapse in women (Scottish Intercollegiate Guidelines Network 2004). Somewhat unusually for NICE guidelines, the Institute will also be considering the competence of surgeons in the field of continence care. These guidelines are due for publication in December 2006.

The role of service users

The Department of Health publication *Good Practice in Continence Services* recommended that service users were involved in the planning, provision and audit of services. This was, at the time, a departure from the usual level of patient involvement in services, often as a mutual support group or not at all involved. As part of the scope for the national audit of continence care for older people, NICE asked that the views of service users be taken in to account and, accordingly, a piece of work to assess the views of service users as to what constitutes quality in services was commissioned by The Royal College of Physicians Clinical Evaluation and Effectiveness Unit. Phase one of this project used qualitative research methods to gauge service users' views based upon the quality standards that were at the time intended to comprise the national audit (Billings & Wagg 2003). The results of this study were then used to create a questionnaire to be used for a wider audience and those items that were rated very important to patients were included in the national audit tool. Interestingly, patients viewed patient support groups as being of low importance to them.

Monitoring the implementation of guidelines and measuring quality

Clinical audit is a difficult process with which to engage on a daily basis and, ideally, it is best conducted when linked to everyday clinical practice, as part of the process of care. Staff time is a major obstacle to carrying out any audit and, although there is funding for audit in all trusts, this is often not the perception of clinical staff who have the task of performing the audit. It is essential that any plans to promote audit in all care settings, especially in the primary care and care home setting, ensure accessible funding that can be applied to support staff in carrying out the work. This is essential to maximise participation in the audit process and to ensure that the findings can be generalised throughout the country.

As part of the monitoring process for the National Service Framework for Older People, the now defunct National Health Service Information Authority has developed and piloted a database for urinary incontinence based upon many of the outcome indicators of care from previous work. These data items will be available within the NHS directory for use by any interested Trust. The return of these data items will not be compulsory for any NHS body, however, and, thus, interest is likely to be low (NHS Health and Social Care Information Centre 2005).

Another way of monitoring standards is to conduct a comparative audit. The Royal College of Physicians Clinical Evaluation and Effectiveness Unit has successfully developed a reliable and robust audit tool for older people which is relevant to people in the community, in hospital and in care home settings and is engaged in the first national audit of practice outside the secondary care environment and breaks new ground in a hitherto under-investigated area of high national priority. The pilot for this project, published in the *Journal of Evaluation in Clinical Practice*, produced interesting results from a limited sample of care settings (Wagg *et al.* 2005). The audit will allow centres direct comparison of their performance compared to quality standards and will inform Primary Care Trusts and independent care organisations with regard to service provision and further development. The tool is applicable to all older people with:

- Lower urinary tract symptoms (voiding and storage disorders)
- Bladder and bowel dysfunction
- Urinary incontinence
- Faecal incontinence
- Constipation

The audit tool includes indicators of:

- Appropriate structures for care including standards relating to personnel, facilities, training programmes and quality maintenance
- Processes for high-quality care including specific requirements for assessment at all entry levels to the system, investigation and treatment
- Recommended clinically relevant outcome measures, including those generated by service users in a wide range of clinical settings
- Clinically relevant measures of the impact of the problem on formal or informal carers
- Quality measures derived by service users and measures of:
- Value for quality maintenance by services
- Case mix, including cognitive and functional status, to allow comparison between sites and settings of care

In a separate though linked project, the views of older service users have been taken into account when considering quality of care and service. The results of this work, modified into measurable standards, have been included in the national audit tool with details published in the *Journal of Evaluation in Clinical Practice* (Mian *et al.* 2005). The audit has been funded by the Healthcare Commission for a cycle of audit, a dissemination and change programme and a subsequent re-audit. Participation in national audits, of which this is one, will be included in the assessment of quality of care by NHS Trusts.

It is clear that the implementation of guidelines produced by national bodies has been patchy across the NHS. NICE is currently embarked upon a revision of its implementation arm with a view to enhancing its role in this area. The requirement for revalidation for practice under the aegis of the General Medical Council, coupled with an increasing governmental, media and public interest in the quality of health care, means that clinical guidelines and monitoring by audit can no longer be ignored or neglected.

Achieving change

The NHS is in a constant cycle of change, aided and abetted by change agents, the (now defunct) Modernisation Agency and a host of other bodies designed to help institutions to redesign how care is delivered. Much work has been focused on areas where there are politically motivated, national performance targets to achieve and this has undoubtedly been effective. The Myocardial Infarction National Audit Project, targets for emergency access and elective procedures have demonstrated the power of centrally mandated, 'must do' performance indicators on the NHS. Such wholesale change has, however, been expensive to achieve and is proving problematic to maintain. The challenge to any clinical effectiveness programme centred around clinical audit is the achievement of meaningful and sustainable change. There are, within the continence field, isolated areas of good practice (Williams *et al.* 2000). What might be achieved in the absence of national directives and without focused funding is less clear. Data feedback alone may in itself be effective, but management of this process needs to be carefully handled to achieve the best response. Feedback depends not only on the quality and timeliness of the data, but also on the perception of the audience as to the purpose of feedback in the context of the organisation. Factors identified as crucial in using data feedback are illustrated in Figure 13.2 (Bradley *et al.* 2004). There is some evidence that comparison of high- and low-performing services may identify variables that are critical to the change process (Cohen *et al.* 2004). However, there is published evidence regarding the generic factors required to achieve change, but there is little evidence of widespread quality improvement, even taking into account the impact of the National Service Framework target of integrated continence services for older people.

- Data must be perceived as valid to motivate change.
- Time is needed to develop the credibility of data.
- The source of data is critical to its perceived validity.
- The feedback should be timely.
- The use of comparative data improves the feedback.
- Data describing individual performance may be perceived as punitive.
- Data feedback must persist to sustain improved performance.

Figure 13.2 Factors associated with a positive outcome from data feedback

Promoting change in clinical services and ensuring sustainability has been the subject of much research with no clear view as to what might be the elements of an effective intervention. Consistent themes from available work appear to be:

1. Motivation of key stakeholders to achieve the target for change
2. Instrumental, personal, and interactive resources for change
3. Motivators outside the service, including the larger health care environment and government
4. Opportunities for change, that is, how key stakeholders understand the change options

Local ownership is an essential requisite for the promotion of any change. Successful change management should be enhanced by use of a framework that includes a clear statement of purpose, stakeholder concordance and trust, clear leadership and structures and fast action together with recognition of achievements. The majority of this evidence comes from other areas of health care and there is still relatively little known about the relative effectiveness of interventions designed to improve the quality of health care or the conditions required to produce a change. Research has been difficult because: interventions change over time, reflecting the dynamics of health care systems; the organisations to which interventions are applied also change; and the national or regional guidelines for services are revised.

There are also data suggesting factors which might lead to the failure of quality improvement programmes, or the failure of the intervention to detect a change (Øvretveit & Gustafson 2003). These appear to be:

* Low levels of participation by sites or stakeholders
* Poorly designed outcome measures
* The difficulty in assigning observed change to the intervention
* The influence of external factors (local health policy, political agenda) on the observed outcome
* The difficulty in separating the influence of each component of the intervention in achieving the change

In addition to local ownership, key opinion leaders within the hospital setting have been shown to be influential in achieving meaningful change in practice (Berner *et al.* 2003), but the sustainability of the achieved improvement has not been assessed in any detail. Several quality outcome indicators are performance based and thus the data items are easily gathered from hospital episode statistics. For example, the rate of anterior vaginal repair for stress incontinence in the absence of prolapse, as suggested by *Good Practice in Continence Services,* should be collectable upon this basis. The use of observational data for new interventions and the creation of 'registers' for new surgical procedures have seldom been adopted to produce data which would have an inherent use for quality measurement, where variance might be highlighted and further analysed to identify areas of good and poor practice.

Conclusion

There has been a proliferation of clinical guidelines in the field of continence care over the past few years. These are now being formalised with the introduction of national guidelines for Scotland and for England and Wales. Where evidence-based guidelines exist, standards or measurable quality measures may be developed against which to compare practice. There needs to be a robust mechanism for monitoring which does not make the collection of the indicators impractical in terms of time and the sparse allocation of central resource for clinical audit. Evidence for clinical audit influencing change in clinical practice and outcome for patients is accumulating, but progress is slow. The additional influence of politically driven targets often acts as a galvanising force to produce change which might otherwise either not occur or only occur slowly. For continence, an area high on the political agenda, but with neither a mandated target other than for the older person, nor additional focused funding, there are techniques that have been proven to induce change in practice and to influence the quality of care in other clinical areas which may be applicable to continence services and their delivery. There is a need for work specifically in continence to test whether these methods are transferable. The national audit is a major step along this pathway.

References

Abrams, P., Cardozo, L., Khoury, S. & Wein, A. (eds) (2005). *Incontinence: Third International Consultation on Incontinence*. Paris: Health Publications Ltd.

AHCPR. (1996). *Urinary Incontinence in Adults, Clinical Practice Guideline Update*. Rockville, MD: Agency for Health Care Policy and Research. Overview: http://www.ahrq.gov/clinic/uiovervw.htm.

Berner, E. S., Baker, C. S., Funkhouser, E., Heudebert, G. R., Allison, J. J., Fargason, C. A. Jr, Li, Q., Person, S. D. & Kiefe, C. I. (2003). Do local opinion leaders augment hospital quality improvement efforts? A randomized trial to promote adherence to unstable angina guidelines. *Medical Care* **41**, 420–431.

Billings, J. & Wagg, A. (2003). *Older Users' Views of Quality Issues in Continence Services. Phase 1. CHSS/Royal College of Physicians Clinical Evaluation and Effectiveness Unit*. London: Royal College of Physicians

Bradley, E. H., Holmboe, E. S., Mattera, J. A., Roumanis, S. A., Radford, M. J. & Krumholz, H. M. (2004). Data feedback efforts in quality improvement: lessons learned from US hospitals. *Quality and Safety in Health Care* **13**, 26–31.

Brocklehurst, J., Amess, M., Goldacre, M., Mason, A., Wilkinson, E., Eastwood, A. & Coles, J. (eds) (1999). *Outcome Indicators for Urinary Incontinence: Report of a National Working Party to the Department of Health*. London: National Centre for Health Outcomes Development.

Button, D., Roe, B., Webb, C., Frith, A., Colin-Thorne, D. & Gardner, L. (1998). *Continence. Promotion and Management by the Primary Health Care Team: Consensus guidelines*. London: Whurr.

Cheater, F., Lakhani, M. & Cawood, C. (1998). *Audit Protocol. Assessment of Patients with Urinary Incontinence*. Leicester: Eli Lily National Clinical Audit Centre.

Cohen, D., McDaniel, R. R. Jr, Crabtree, B. F., Ruhe, M. C., Weyer, S. M., Tallia, A., Miller, W. L., Goodwin, M. A., Nutting, P., Solberg, L. I. *et al.* (2004). A practice change model for quality improvement in primary care practice. *Journal of Health Care Management* **49**, 155–168.

Cranney, M., Barton, S. & Walley, T. (1999). Addressing barriers to change: an RCT of practice-based education to improve management of hypertension in the elderly. *British Journal of General Practice* **49**, 522–526.

Department of Health. (1998a). *A First Class Service: Quality in the New NHS.* London: Department of Health.

Department of Health. (1998b). *The New NHS: Modern and Dependable. A National Framework for Assessing Performance Consultation Document, EL (98)4.* London: Department of Health.

Department of Health. (2000). *Good Practice in Continence Services.* London: Department of Health.

Eustice, S., Roe, B. & Paterson, J. (2005). Prompted voiding for the management of urinary incontinence in adults (Cochrane review) 2000. *The Cochrane Library*, issue 3. Chichester: Wiley. http://www.update-software.com/Abstracts/ab002113.htm.

Feder, G., Griffiths, C., Highton, C., Eldridge, S., Spence, M. & Southgate, L. (1995). Do clinical guidelines introduced with practice based education improve care of asthmatics and diabetic patients? A randomised controlled trial in general practice in east London. *British Medical Journal* **311**, 1473–1478.

Georgiou, A., Potter, J. M., Brocklehurst, J., Lowe, D. & Pearson, M. (2001). Measuring the quality of continence care in long term care facilities: an analysis of outcome indicators. *Age and Ageing* **30**, 63–66.

Hampel, C., Hohenfellner, M., Abrams, P., Andersen, J. T., Chartier-Castler, E. J., Tammela, T. L. J., van Kerrebroeck, P., Vignoli, G. & Thüroff, J. W. (1999). *Guidelines on Incontinence.* European Association of Urology. http://www.woweb.nl/files/uploaded_files/2001_incontinence.pdf.

Hay-Smith, J., Herbison, P. & Mørkved, S. (2005). Physical therapies for prevention of urinary and faecal incontinence in adults (Cochrane review) 2003. *The Cochrane Library*, issue 3. Chichester: Wiley. http://www.update-software.com/Abstracts/ab003191.htm.

Irwin, P., Hoffman, A., Lowe, D., Pearson, M. G. & Rudd, A. G. (2005). Improving clinical practice in stroke through audit: results of three rounds of National Stroke Audit. *Journal of Evaluation in Clinical Practice* **11**, 306–314.

Mian, S., Wagg, A., Potter, J., Irwin, P. & Pearson, M. (2005). National audit of continence care for older people: resources and method. *Journal of Evaluation in Clinical Practice* **11**, 533–543.

National Service Framework for Older People. (2001). London: Department of Health.

NHS Health and Social Care Information Centre. (2005). *Datasets Development.* http://www.icservices.nhs.uk/datasets/pages/continence.asp (accessed 8 August 2005).

Øvretveit, J. & Gustafson, D. (2003). Using research to inform quality programmes. *British Medical Journal* **326**, 759–761.

Research Unit, Royal College of Physicians of London. (1998). *Promoting Continence: Clinical Audit Scheme for the Management of Urinary and Faecal Incontinence.* London: Royal College of Physicians of London.

Royal College of Nursing. (2000). *The Essence of Care: Patient-focused Benchmarking for Health Care Practitioners.* London: Department of Health.

Royal College of Physicians of London. (1998). *The CARE Scheme (Continuous Assessment Review and Evaluation): Clinical Audit of Long-term Care of Elderly People*, 2nd edn. London: Royal College of Physicians of London.

Royal College of Physicians of London. (2000). *The Health and Care of Older People in Care Homes. A Comprehensive Interdisciplinary Approach: Report of a Joint Working Party of the Royal College of Physicians, the Royal College of Nursing and the British Geriatrics Society*. London: Royal College of Physicians.

Scottish Intercollegiate Guidelines Network. (2004). *Management of Urinary Incontinence in Primary Care: A National Clinical Guideline*. http://www.sign.ac.uk/guidelines/published/index.html#Other.

Thomas, S. (2003). *Is Policy Translated into Action?* London: Continence Foundation.

Wagg, A., Mian, S., Lowe, D., Potter, J. & Pearson, M. (2005). The national audit of continence care for older people: results of a pilot study. *Journal of Evaluation in Clinical Practice*. **11**, 525–532.

Wallace, S. A., Roe, B., Williams, K. & Palmer, M. (2005). Bladder training for urinary incontinence in adults (Cochrane review) 2003. *The Cochrane Library*, issue 3. Chichester: Wiley. http://www.update-software.com/Abstracts/ab001308.htm.

Williams, K. S., Assassa, R. P., Smith, N. K., Jagger, C., Perry, S., Shaw, C., Dallosso, H., McGrother, C., Clarke, M., Brittain, K. R. *et al.* (2000). Development, implementation and evaluation of a new nurse continence service: a pilot study. *Journal of Clinical Nursing* **9**, 566–573.

Working Group on Outcome Indicators for Urinary Incontinence. (1997). *National Centre for Health Outcomes Development Report to the Department of Health*. London, UK.

Chapter 14

Quality of life and lower urinary tract dysfunction

Dudley Robinson and Linda Cardozo

Introduction

Urinary incontinence is a distressing and disabling condition causing significant morbidity within society in addition to affecting the social, psychological, occupational, domestic, physical and sexual lives of 15–30% of women of all ages (Thomas *et al.* 1980). Although it remains a cause of substantial morbidity, comparable to other chronic disease processes (Figure 14.1), over 50% of incontinent women never seek help for their condition (Norton *et al.* 1988), thus the prevalence is often underestimated.

Research has often concentrated on the prevalence, aetiology, diagnosis and management of urinary incontinence with little work being performed on the effects of this chronic condition, or its treatment, on quality of life (QoL). Over the past few decades interest in the incorporation of patient assessed health status or QoL measures into the evaluation of the management of urinary incontinence has increased (Fitzpatrick *et al.* 1992).

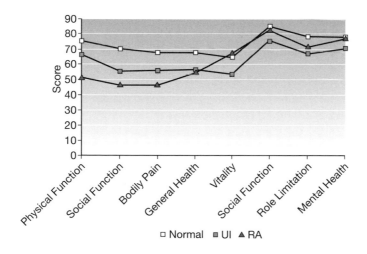

Figure 14.1 Short form 36 scores: Comparison to other diseases. Urge urinary incontinence [UI], rheumatoid arthritis [RA], and normals

The views of clinicians and patients about QoL and the effects of treatments differ considerably. Consequently, there is increased recognition of the patient's perception when assessing new interventions in the management of lower urinary tract dysfunction. The measurement of QoL allows the quantification of morbidity, the evaluation of treatment efficacy and also acts as a measure of how lives are affected and coping strategies adopted. It is estimated that 20% of adult women suffer some degree of life disruption secondary to lower urinary tract dysfunction (Burgio *et al.* 1991).

Quality of life

The World Health Organization (WHO 1978) has defined health as 'not merely the absence of disease, but complete physical, mental and social wellbeing'. Quality of life has been used to mean a combination of patient assessed measures of health including physical function, role function, social function, emotional or mental state, burden of symptoms and sense of wellbeing (Coulter 1993). QoL has been defined as including 'those attributes valued by patients including their resultant comfort or sense of well being; the extent to which they were able to maintain reasonable physical, emotional, and intellectual function; the degree to which they retain their ability to participate in valued activities within the family and the community' (Naughton *et al.* 1996). This helps to emphasise the multidimensional nature of QoL and the importance of considering patients perception of their own situation with regard to non-health related aspects of their life (Gill *et al.* 1974).

Although quality of life is highly subjective, it has now been acknowledged that it is as important as physical disease state in the management of women with lower urinary tract dysfunction (Murawaski 1978). Consequently, the success of treatment can no longer be judged on clinical parameters alone and quality of life needs to be considered in both clinical and research settings (Blavis *et al.* 1997) (Table 14.1).

Table 14.1 Applications of quality of life questionnaires

Screening and monitoring for psychosocial problems in patient care
Population surveys of perceived health problems
Study the effect of disease processes on the individual
Evaluation of intervention on the disease process
Medical audit
Outcome measures in health services
Clinical trials
Cost-utility analysis
Adjunct to the consultation

Assessment of quality of life

There are many validated questionnaires available although all have the same structure, consisting of a series of sections (domains) designed to gather information regarding particular aspects of health (Table 14.2). There are two types of QoL questionnaires, generic and disease, or condition specific.

More recently, the International Consultation on Incontinence (ICI) has published levels of recommendation for both generic and disease-specific questionnaires (Donovan *et al.* 2002) (Table 14.3).

Table 14.2 Quality of life domains

Physical function, e.g. mobility, self care, exercise

Emotional function, e.g. depression, anxiety, worry

Social function, e.g. intimacy, social support, social contact leisure activities

Role performance, e.g. work, housework, shopping

Pain

Sleep/nausea

Disease-specific symptoms

Severity measures

Table 14.3 Criteria for the recommendation of questionnaires

Grade of recommendation	*Evidence required*
Grade A Highly recommended	Published data indicating that it is valid, reliable and responsive to change on psychometric testing
Grade B Recommended	Published data indicating that it is valid and reliable on psychometric testing
Grade C With potential	Published data (including abstracts) indicating that it is valid or reliable or responsive on psychometric testing

Generic quality of life questionnaires

Generic questionnaires are designed as general measures of QoL and are therefore applicable to a wide range of populations and clinical conditions. Many different validated generic questionnaires have been developed although not all are suitable for the assessment of lower urinary tract problems (Table 14.4). They are not specific to a particular disease, treatment or age group and hence allow broad comparisons to be made. Consequently, they lack sensitivity when applied to women with lower urinary tract symptoms and may be unable to detect clinically important improvement.

Table 14.4 Generic quality of life questionnaires

Generic Quality of Life Questionnaires (Grade A) Short Form 36 (SF-36) (Lyons *et al.* 1994)
Generic Quality of Life Questionnaires (Grade B) Sickness Impact Profile (Hunskaar & Vinsnes 1991) Nottingham Health Profile (Grimby *et al.* 1993) Goteborg Quality of Life (Sullivan *et al.* 1993)

Disease-specific quality of life questionnaires

To improve the sensitivity of QoL questionnaires, disease-specific tools have been developed to assess particular medical conditions more accurately and in greater detail (Table 14.5). The questions are designed to focus on key aspects associated with lower urinary tract symptoms while scoring is performed so that clinically important changes can be detected.

In general, perhaps the best solution when assessing women with urinary incontinence is to use a generic and a disease-specific questionnaire in combination, both of which have been validated and used previously.

Table 14.5 Disease-specific quality of life questionnaires

Urogenital Distress Inventory (UDI) (Shumaker *et al.* 1994) Urogenital Distress Inventory – 6 (UDI-6) (Uebersax *et al.* 1995) Urge UDI (Lubeck *et al.* 1999) Incontinence Severity Index (Sandvik *et al.* 1993) Quality of life in persons with urinary incontinence (I-QoL) (Wagner *et al.* 1996) King's Health Questionnaire (Kelleher *et al.* 1997) Incontinence Impact Questionnaire (IIQ) (Wyman *et al.* 1987)

Assessment of urinary symptoms

Although urinary incontinence is known to result in impairment of quality of life this is difficult to predict, using symptoms and urodynamic studies alone. Different individuals vary greatly in their perception of incontinence and QoL questionnaires are useful in objectively assessing the impact of lower urinary tract dysfunction.

In clinical practice, urinary symptoms alone may be inaccurate in diagnosing lower urinary tract dysfunction (Bergman & Bader 1990; Versi *et al.* 1991). When comparing the results of clinical and urodynamic assessment in 100 women there was agreement in 68% of cases of urodynamic stress incontinence and only 51% of cases of detrusor overactivity. 46% of those women with urodynamic stress incontinence also complained of urgency, whereas 26% of those women with detrusor overactivity complained of stress incontinence (Jarvis *et al.* 1980). The symptom of stress incontinence in the absence of urge incontinence has been shown to have a sensitivity of 78%, specificity of 84% and positive predictive value of 87% (Lagro-Jansson *et al.* 1991), whereas if stress incontinence is the only reported symptom then the diagnosis is likely to be urodynamic stress incontinence in over 90% of cases (Farrar *et al.* 1975). In addition, there is little correlation between objective loss during pad testing and subjective assessment using visual analogue scores (Fraser *et al.* 1989).

In general, there is only a poor relationship between subjective assessment and objective urodynamic diagnosis limiting the usefulness of symptom questionnaires alone. QoL questionnaires are therefore a useful adjunct, helping to assess the impact of urinary incontinence and bladder dysfunction.

Urinary symptoms and quality of life

Many studies have been performed examining the effect of lower urinary tract dysfunction, especially incontinence, on quality of life, although there is a wide variation in study design and methodology. Early studies using symptom questionnaires to estimate the prevalence of urinary symptoms have demonstrated the effects of restriction of activities and also the financial burden of urinary incontinence.

Scoring systems have been developed to examine the effects of incontinence on QoL, including sexual problems and embarrassment, although the degree of incontinence did not correlate with the degree of disability (Norton 1982).

Sexual function

The effect of urinary incontinence in relation to sexual function has also been investigated. In a study of women attending an incontinence clinic, 46% felt that their urinary symptoms affected sexual function. Those women with detrusor overactivity had a significantly higher incidence of sexual dysfunction than those with urodynamic stress incontinence (Sutherst 1979). A comparison of sexual function in women with and without urogenital prolapse and urinary incontinence has also been performed. Measures of sexual function did not differ between the two groups and a similar proportion of women were sexually active. Interest in sexual activity was unchanged in 70% of women and 84% reported satisfaction. 44% of sexually active women with prolapse admitted to urinary incontinence during intercourse whereas 31% felt that incontinence or prolapse interfered with sexual activity. The authors concluded that women with urogenital prolapse and urinary incontinence are not different from controls in measures of sexual function and age is the most important factor predicting sexual activity (Weber *et al.* 1995).

Psychosocial function

To examine the psychosocial impact of urinary incontinence, 69 community dwelling women were assessed using the Incontinence Impact Questionnaire in addition to undergoing urodynamic evaluation and completing urinary dairies and a pad test.

Those women with detrusor overactivity, with or without concomitant sphincter incompetence, reported significantly higher impact scores than those with sphincter incompetence alone. In addition, there was a correlation between psychosocial impact scores and the severity of incontinence (Wyman *et al.* 1987).

More recently, a large community-based study in Austria has been performed examining the impact of urinary incontinence in the general population using the Bristol Female Lower Urinary Tract Symptoms Score (BFLUTS). Prevalence increased with age and, overall, 65.7% of women felt their Quality of Life was impaired by their incontinence. Patient age and duration of symptoms had no significant effect on impairment of quality of life although frequency and degree of incontinence, impact on sexual function and need for incontinence devices were found to have a significant effect. Additionally, 25.1% complained of sexual dysfunction (Temml *et al.* 2000). A postal survey of 2075 women in the UK revealed some degree of incontinence in 69% of women during the previous month although only 30% felt it had social or hygienic impact. The most troublesome symptoms were found to be incontinence for no obvious reason, nocturnal incontinence and nocturia (Swithinbank *et al.* 1999).

Age

Little is known about the effect of age on the subjective severity of incontinence. In a sample of elderly women complaining of genitourinary problems, 72% thought their symptoms were normal at their age (Gjorp *et al.* 1987). A further community based study of 1442 women in The Netherlands supports these findings. Overall, 22.5% of women complained of urinary incontinence, although 77.8% were not concerned and 75.4% did not feel restricted in their activities. When considering severe incontinence, only 15.6% were concerned and 15.7% restricted their activities. Interestingly, only one third had been identified by their general practitioner as having a significant problem (Lagro-Janssen *et al.* 1990). This may explain why the elderly tend to present later for the assessment and treatment of lower urinary tract dysfunction (Norton *et al.* 1988).

More recently, the effect of age on Quality of Life impairment has been investigated. Using the Sickness Impact Profile (SIP), 36 women aged between 40 and 60 from an incontinence clinic were assessed. Psychosocial and physical dysfunction was found in 7% and 8% of the women, respectively, with urge symptoms being associated with more impairment than those of stress incontinence. Those with the symptom of stress incontinence were relatively little affected whereas the younger women were affected severely. This was most evident when examining emotional behaviour, recreation and pastimes (Hunskaar & Vinsnes 1992). Similar findings were reported when comparing a group of elderly patients suffering from urinary incontinence with an age matched control group using the Nottingham Health Profile (NHP). Women with incontinence obtained higher scores in the domains of emotional disturbances and social isolation when compared to the control group. Those with urge or mixed incontinence reported a higher degree of emotional disturbance and sleep disturbance than those in the control group, although this difference was not seen in those complaining of stress incontinence (Grimby *et al.* 1993).

The effect of urinary symptoms around the time of the menopause has also recently been investigated in a Danish ongoing longitudinal cohort study of 4000 women between the ages of 40 and 60 years old using a self administered questionnaire: 27.8% of women complained of lower urinary tract symptoms. There was an age related increase in both urge and stress incontinence. Age was associated with symptoms, although not with bothersomeness, whereas urinary symptoms occurring more often than once per week were the best indicator of lower urinary tract dysfunction (Moller *et al.* 2000).

The King's Health Questionnaire

The King's Health Questionnaire (KHQ) was developed in the department of Urogynaecology at King's College Hospital (Kelleher *et al.* 1997). Between 1991 and 1993, 1105 consecutive women referred with lower urinary tract symptoms were asked to complete a generic QoL questionnaire in addition to a detailed disease-specific questionnaire relating to urinary incontinence. The questions were devised from previously published generic and disease-specific QoL questionnaires following discussion with women themselves. Six pilot versions were used, the final draft having 21 questions in eight different domains and a separate scale for measuring the severity of urinary symptoms (Table 14.6). A four-point scoring system was used for each of the items and included an inapplicable option for questions relating to personal relationships to enable all women to answer each item. Each of the domains is scored in a similar way and thus each contributes similarly to the overall score. Scores in each domain range between 0 and 100, a higher score indicating a greater impairment of quality of life. The final version was then mailed to 293 consecutive women referred for urodynamic investigation.

Internal reliability was assessed using Cronbach's alpha statistic whereas test–retest reliability was assessed by asking 110 women chosen at random to complete the questionnaire a second time. Both confirmed a high degree of reproducibility. Criterion validity was then tested by measuring the correlation of the King's QoL scores with those obtained using the UK version Short Form 36 in a subgroup of 193 women. Although not all domains are common to both of these instruments, there was a highly significant correlation in those that are.

The KHQ is easy to complete, valid and a reliable instrument for the assessment of women with urinary incontinence, so it continues to be used for clinical and research purposes. In addition, it has been used in many major clinical trials and has now been modified for a number of different cultures and languages. It has been translated into a total of 34 languages including French, German, Greek, Spanish,

Table 14.6 Domains of the King's Health Questionnaire

Part I
General health perception
Incontinence impact
Part II
Role limitations
Physical limitations
Social limitations
Personal relationships
Emotions
Severity measures
Part III
Disease-specific questions; frequency, nocturia, urgency, urge incontinence, stress incontinence, nocturnal enuresis, intercourse incontinence, infections, pain, difficulty in voiding

Swiss, Italian, French and English Canadian and US English, and has been validated in men (Kobelt *et al.* 1999).

Experience using the KHQ has shown that over 70% of women with urodynamic stress incontinence, detrusor overactivity, low compliance, mixed incontinence and normal urodynamics considered their health to be fair or better than normal, whereas those with sensory urgency reported worse overall health. However, incontinence impact scores were significantly worse for those women with detrusor overactivity than with urodynamic stress incontinence (Figure 14.2) and significantly better in those women with normal urodynamics. In addition, when considering the separate health domains women with detrusor overactivity had significantly more impairment to quality of life in all domains except physical limitations when compared to those with urodynamic stress incontinence (Figure 14.3). Interestingly, the perception of severity of urinary incontinence was greater in women with urodynamic stress incontinence than detrusor overactivity, although this did not reach significance.

More recently, the KHQ has been used to assess the subjective and objective outcomes following primary and repeat colposuspension (Bidmead *et al.* 2001). Objective results of surgery were assessed with repeat videocystourethrography 6–12 months after surgery, whereas subjective results were evaluated using a condition specific QoL tool, KHQ. Symptom severity was also evaluated as a component of the condition specific QoL questionnaire.

Objective cure was demonstrated in 92% of women undergoing primary surgery with an 8% incidence of *de novo* detrusor overactivity and a 10% incidence of voiding difficulties. In the group of women having repeat surgery, the objective cure rate was 81% with no *de novo* detrusor overactivity and a 6% incidence of postoperative voiding difficulties. QoL scores improved in 95% of women. Improvements of over

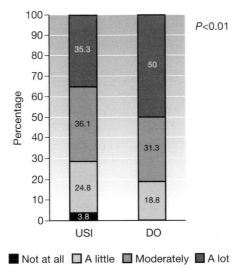

Figure 14.2 Effect of bladder symptoms on quality of life

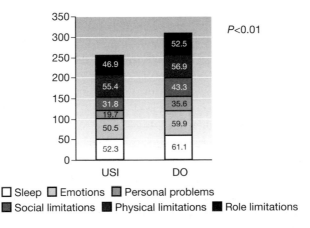

Figure 14.3 Quality of life scores and urodynamics diagnosis

25% were seen in 70% of women and of over 50% in 28%. Changes in the scores for the eight quality of life domains were also analysed. Improvements were seen in all domains other than general health perception. Statistical analysis using Wilcoxon ranked pairs test showed highly significant improvements in all of these domains. This would support previous studies investigating quality of life following continence surgery (Kondo *et al.* 1992).

Deterioration in QoL scores was recorded by 2.4% of women. This represented two women, one of whom was troubled by persistent irritive urinary symptoms after surgery whereas the other complained of chronic lower abdominal discomfort, thought to be related to the colposuspension sutures.

Objectively, 11 women had persistent stress incontinence on post colposuspension urodynamic testing. Conventionally, these women would be regarded as having had failed surgery. Closer examination of the results of QoL assessment for these women shows significant improvement in QoL scores in this group. This compares favourably with the improvement in scores in the group with cure of stress incontinence on urodynamic testing. These results highlight the fact that while objective testing may be important in defining the outcome of surgery it can give a false impression of the symptomatic results and women who have persistent stress incontinence during cystometry may not, in fact, be symptomatic during daily life.

Conclusion

Quality of life questionnaires have been shown to be a useful adjunct in the investigation and management of women with lower urinary tract dysfunction complimenting standard investigations such as urodynamics and pad testing. They provide an objective measure of the impact of incontinence which is essential to the accurate investigation and evaluation of patients and new treatment protocols. In addition, they have an important role in research, both in pharmacological and surgical trials, and in audit activities, allowing accurate assessment of new and established treatments and their impact on quality of life.

References

Bergman, A. & Bader, K. (1990). Reliability of the patient's history in the diagnosis of urinary incontinence. *International Journal of Gynaecology and Obstetrics* **32**, 255–259.

Bidmead, J., Cardozo, L., McLellan, A., Khullar, V. & Kelleher, C. (2001). A Comparison of the objective and subjective outcomes of colposuspension for stress incontinence in women. *British Journal of Obstetrics and Gynaecology* **108**, 408–413.

Blavis, J. G., Appell, R. A., Fantl, J. A. *et al.* (1997). Standards of efficacy for evaluation of treatment outcomes in urinary incontinence: recommendations of the urodynamics society. *Neurourology and Urodynamics* **16**, 145–147.

Burgio, K. L., Matthews, K. A. & Engel, B. T. (1991). Prevalence, incidence and correlates of urinary incontinence in healthy, middle-aged women. *Journal of Urology* **146**, 1255–1259.

Coulter, A. (1993). Measuring quality of life. In *Critical Reading in General Practice* (ed. A. L. Kinmouth & R. Jones). Oxford: Oxford University Press.

Donovan, J. L., Badia, X., Corcos, J., Gotoh, M., Kelleher, C. J., Naughton, M. & Shaw, C. (2002). Symptom and quality of life assessment. In *Incontinence*, 2nd edition (ed. P. Abrams, L. Cardozo, S. Khoury & A. Wein), pp. 267–316. Plymouth, UK: Health Publication.

Farrar, D. J., Whiteside, C. G., Osbourne, J. L. & Turner-Warwick R. T. (1975). A urodynamic analysis of micturition symptoms in the female. *Surgery, Gynecology and Obstetrics* **141**, 875–881.

Fitzpatrick, R., Fletcher, A., Gore, S., Jones, D., Spiegelhalter, D. & Cox, D. (1992). Quality of life measures in healthcare. 1: Applications and issues in assessment. *British Medical Journal* **305**, 1075–1077.

Fraser, M. I., Haylen, B. T. & Suthherst, J. R. (1989). The severity of urinary incontinence in women. Comparison of subjective and objective tests. *British Journal of Urology* **63**, 14–15.

Gill, T. M. & Feinstein, A. R. (1974). A critical appraisal of the quality of life measurements. *Journal of the American Medical Association* **272**, 619–626.

Gjorp, T., Hendriksen, C., Lund, E. & Stromgard, E. (1987). Is growing old a disease? A study of the attitudes of elderly people to physical symptoms. *Journal of Chronic Diseases* **40** 1095–1098.

Grimby, A., Milsom, I., Molander, U., Wiklund, I. & Ekelund P. (1993). The influence of urinary incontinence on the quality of life of elderly women. *Age and Aging* **22**, 82–89.

Hunskaar, S. & Vinsnes, A. (1991). The quality of life in women with urinary incontinence as measured by the sickness impact profile. *Journal of the American Geriatrics Society* **39**, 378–382.

Jarvis, G. J., Hall, S., Stamp, S., Millar, D. R. & Johnson, A. (1980). An assessment of urodynamic examination in incontinent women. *British Journal of Obstetrics and Gynaecology*; **87**, 893–896.

Kelleher, C. J., Cardozo, L. D., Khullar, V. & Salvatore, S. (1997). A new questionnaire to assess the quality of life of urinary incontinent women. *British Journal of Obstetrics and Gynaecology* **104**, 1374–1379.

Kobelt, G., Kirchberger, I. & Malone–Lee, J. (1999). Quality of life aspects of the overactive bladder and the effect of treatment with Tolterodine. *BJU International* **83**, 583–590.

Kondo, A., Itoh, Y., Yamada, M., Saito, M. & Kato, K. (1992). Effects of urinary incontinence on quality of life. *International Urogynecology Journal* **3**, 121–123.

Lagro-Janssen, T. L., Smits, A. J. & Van Weel, C. (1990). Women with urinary incontinence: self-percieved worries and general practitioners' knowledge of the problem. *British Journal of General Practice* **40**, 331–334.

Lagro-Jansson, A. L., Debruyne, F. M. & Van Weel, C. (1991). Value of patients case history in diagnosing urinary incontinence in general practice. *British Journal of Urology* **67**, 569–572.

Lubeck, D. P., Prebil, L. A., Peebles, P. & Brown, J. S. (1999). A health related quality of life measure for use in patients with urge urinary incontinence: a validation study. *Quality of Life Research* **8**, 337–344.

Lyons, R. A., Perry, H. M. & Littlepage, B. N. C. (1994). Evidence for the validity of the short form 36 questionnaire (SF-36) in an elderly population. *Age and Ageing* **23**, 182–184.

Moller, L. A., Lose, G. & Jorgensen, T. (2000). The prevalence and bothersomeness of lower urinary tract symptoms in women 40-60 years of age. *Acta Obstetricia et Gynecologica Scandinavica* **79**, 298–305.

Murawaski, B. J. (1978). Social support in health and illness; the concept and its measurement. *Canadian Nurse* **1**, 365–371.

Naughton, M. J. & Shumaker, S. A. (1996). Assessment of health related quality of life. In *Fundamentals of clinical trials*, 3rd edition (ed. C. D. Furberg, & D. L. DeMets), p. 185. St Louis: Mosby Press.

Norton, C. (1982). The effects of urinary incontinence in women. *International Rehabilitation Medicine* **4**, 9–14.

Norton, P. A., MacDonald, L. D., Sedgwick, P. M. & Stanton, S. L. (1988). Distress and delay associated with urinary incontinence, frequency and urgency in women. *British Medical Journal* **297**, 1187–1189.

Sandvik, H., Hunskaar, S., Seim, A., Hermstad, R., Vanik, A. & Bratt, H. (1993). Validation of a severity index in female urinary incontinence and its implementation in an epidemiological survey. *Journal of Epidemiology and Community Health Medicine* **47**, 497–499.

Shumaker, S. A., Wyman, J. F., Uebersax, J. S., McClish, D. & Fantl, J.A. (1994). Health related quality of life measures for women with urinary incontinence: the Incontinence Impact Questionnaire and the urogenital distress inventory. *Quality of Life Research* **3**, 291–306.

Sullivan, M., Karlsson, J., Bengtsson, C., Furunes, B., Lapidus, L. & Lissner, L. (1993). The Goteberg Quality of life instrument – A psychometric evaluation of assessments of symptoms and well being among women in a general population. *Scandinavian Journal of Primary Health Care* **11**, 267–275.

Sutherst, J. R. (1979). Sexual dysfunction and urinary incontinence. *British Journal of Obstetrics and Gynaecology* **86**, 387–388.

Swithinbank, L. V., Donovan, J. l., du Heaume, J. C., Rogers, C. A., James, M. C., Yang, Q. & Abrams, P. (1999). Urinary symptoms and incontinence in women: relationships between occurrence, age and perceived impact. *British Journal of General Practice* **49**, 897–900.

Temml, C., Haidinger, G., Schmidbauer, J., Schatzl, G. & Madersbacher, S. (2000). Urinary incontinence in both sexes: prevalence rates and impact on quality of life and sexual life. *Neurourology and Urodynamics* **19**, 259–271.

Thomas, T. M., Plymat, K. R., Blannin, J. & Meade, T.W. (1980). Prevalence of urinary incontinence. *British Medical Journal* **281**, 1243–1245.

Uebersax, J. S., Wyman, J. F., Shumaker, S. A., McClish, D. K. & Fantl, A. J. (1995) Short forms to assess life quality and symptom distress for urinary incontinence in women; The incontinence impact questionnaire and the urogenital distress inventory. *Neurourology and Urodynamics* **14**, 131–139.

Versi, E., Cardozo, L., Anand, D. & Cooper, D. (1991). Symptoms analysis for the diagnosis of genuine stress incontinence. 1991. *British Journal of Obstetrics and Gynaecology* **98**, 815–819.

Wagner, T. H., Patrick, D. L., Bavendam, T. G., Martin, M. L., Buesching, D. P. (1996). Quality of life of persons with urinary incontinence: development of a new measure. *Urology* **47** 67–72.

Weber, A. M., Walters, M. D., Schover, L. R. & Mitchinson, A. (1995). Sexual function in women with urogenital prolapse and urinary incontinence. *Obstetrics and Gynecology* **85**, 483–487.

World Health Organization. (1978). Definition of health from preamble to the constitution of the WHO basic documents, 28th edition. Geneva: WHO.

Wyman, J. F., Harkins, S. W., Choi, S. C., Taylor, J. R. & Fantl, J. A. (1987). Psychosocial impact of incontinence in women. *Obstetrics and Gynecology* **70**, 378–381.

Index